Radiant Body, Restful Mind

Radiant Body, Restful Mind

A Woman's Book of Comfort

Shubhra Krishan

NEW WORLD LIBRARY
NOVATO, CALIFORNIA

New World Library
14 Pamaron Way
Novato, California 94949

Copyright © 2004 by Shubhra Krishan

Edited by Katharine Farnam Conolly
Cover design by Mary Ann Casler
Text design and typography by Cathey Flickinger

The material in this book is intended for education. It is not meant to take the place
of diagnosis and treatment by a qualified medical practitioner or therapist.
No expressed or implied guarantee as to the effects of the use of the
recommendations can be given nor liability taken.

Library of Congress Cataloging-in-Publication Data
Krishan, Shubhra.
Radiant body, restful mind : a woman's book of comfort /
Shubhra Krishan
p.   cm.
ISBN 1-57731-421-2 (paperback : alk. paper)
1. Women—Health and hygiene—popular works.   2. Self-care, Health—Popular
works. I. Title.
RA778.K75   2004
613'.04244—dc22   2003 025215

First printing, March 2004
ISBN 1-57731-421-2
Printed in Canada on 100% postconsumer waste recycled paper
Distributed to the trade by Publishers Group West

10 9 8 7 6 5 4 3 2 1

To my father,
who was everything I want to be.

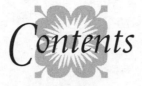Contents

Acknowledgments

I AM DEEPLY GRATEFUL TO:

Georgia Hughes, for placing her trust in me yet again.

Katie Farnam Conolly, gentle yet firm, the guiding light of this book.

My husband, Hemant, who is always just an unspoken whisper away when I need him.

My brother Sachin, whose dreams for me are my inspiration.

My son Harshvardhan, who cheerfully sacrificed several outings because I was busy with the book!

Hannah Polmer, for helping me connect with several women quoted in this book.

All my family members and friends who contributed their tips and ideas to this work.

Most of all, to my mother, for her unconditional love.

Introduction

*L*ife offers you two kinds of simple pleasures. Those that you get for free, as perks for being part of this beautiful world: the scent of rain, a fresh breeze, wildflowers, love. Then there are the pleasures that you create for yourself, simply by taking the time: a rejuvenating walk, a warm bath, tea with a friend on a summer afternoon.

It is about these self-made pleasures that I write here. I've seen that taking the time to savor them can take your body from weary to radiant, your mind from restive to restful, and your life from humdrum to humming. Like little rest-stops along the highway of life, these gifts of kindness to yourself can make the journey a more positive, pleasurable one.

Take a moment to sample some delectable life-enriching ideas with me:

- When you're feeling blue, pick up a family album and travel back through the times when life was uncomplicated and you were happy. You will feel your mood lift.

- Go ahead — take a nap. Just for fifteen minutes, sleep like a dozen logs. You'll wake up feeling like you can make magic.

- Keep a pitcher filled with iced tea or pure mineral water in your refrigerator for a sip of instant bliss.

Like a bee flitting from flower to flower in search of the sweetest nectar, I've spent twenty delicious years seeking such recipes for comfort. I've culled them from meadows far and wide — magazines, books, people, places, words, and moments — and all along, it has been an immensely pleasurable quest.

But wait. A bee's hunt doesn't end with what it finds.

When a scout bee finds the right flower, she performs a special dance for the other honeybees, inviting them to delve inside the petals of a waiting flower, ripe with sunshine and juice.

This book is my dance for you. Between its pages, you'll find life-enhancing secrets I've gathered and treasured. Take time to try any, some, or all of these ideas — not just because I'm urging you to, but because you'd love to, you have been longing to, and you totally deserve to.

I promise you'll find them bee-licious.

CHAPTER I

Joie de Vivre

How to Enjoy and Energize the Body You Inhabit

The human body is not a thing or a substance,
given, but a continuous creation . . .
— NORMAN O. BROWN

As a kid-rearing, hair-tearing, bus-hopping, word-chopping, seldom-stopping, coffee-drinking, hardly-blinking big-city girl, I can relate to hectic lifestyles. But wait. Does that mean I've resigned myself to a lifetime of self-neglect? No way! Not when I'm armed with a powerful secret for looking and feeling bright even on a high-voltage Monday packed with deadlines.

Usually I'm good at keeping secrets, but this one is too delectable not to be shared aloud. So here it is: I tweak time. Don't get me wrong. I don't shirk work or compromise on its quality. In fact, my boss knows about and appreciates my self-improvement strategy. All I do is help myself to a little me-minute here and a few self-care-seconds there — tiny crumbs of time sprinkled throughout my day. For a long time, I didn't even realize how many of these "crumbs" I had available to me that I let slip through my fingers — like the stray dollars I spent on a cup of coffee, a phone call, or a greeting card. Then, out of sheer desperation to perk up my ever-plummeting energy levels, I started noticing the tiny treasures of time that were begging for me to spot and use them.

To my surprise, I found a bounty of "free" time in my day — minutes and seconds that seemed to be pleading "pick me up for a pick-me-up!" Here's a sampling:

Five minutes in the morning, just before getting out of bed.

Perfect for breathing deeply, stretching lightly, and thinking positive thoughts.

Sixty minutes while driving to work and back.

Wonderful for listening to soothing music, singing to myself, breathing deeply at traffic lights, relaxing my death-grip on the steering wheel, and practicing butt-squeezes and Kegel exercises. (To learn the basic Kegel exercise, which tones the muscles of the pelvic floor, see sidebar.)

Fifteen minutes of tea-break at work.

Great for a walk up and down the office corridor, sipping a restorative cup of herb tea, or taking a few minutes to meditate — instead of indulging in idle office gossip.

The fifteen-minute midday slump that nearly always hits after lunch.

Just right for a quick trip to the restroom to give my hair a wake-me-up combing and my mouth a refreshing rinse, or for practicing gentle yoga poses.

Five-to-ten-minute-morsels in the kitchen, while waiting for food to cook.

Ideal for on-the-spot jogging, whipping up a skin-relief pack with ingredients being used in cooking, or thinking up quick, creative ways to add more flavor and health to a dish (read on for ideas!).

At least five three-minute chunks during commercial breaks on television.

Terrific for a few posture-correcting exercises, spritzing cool water on my face, or simply resting my eyes by closing them lightly.

Ten to fifteen minutes while talking on the phone.

Splendid for walking tall as I talk (no tucking the receiver between my shoulder and ear), lightly kneading my back and shoulders with my free hand, or sipping a glass of water as I listen to the person on the other end.

Five to ten minutes at night, in bed, waiting for sleep to steal in.

The perfect time for breathing deeply, visualizing the day's

HOW TO DO THE KEGEL EXERCISE

Named after Dr. Arnold Kegel, the man who developed it, the Kegel exercise is easy to do any time, anywhere, without anyone noticing you. Done regularly, it strengthens the pelvic floor, preventing incontinence and prolapse of the bladder and uterus. Bonus: Strong vaginal muscles enhance sexual pleasure for both you and your partner.

1. Locate your pelvic floor muscles by trying to stop the flow of urine midway, just briefly. The muscles you feel contracting at this point are the muscles you need to exercise.

2. Simply squeeze and release the muscles between twenty-five and fifty times.

3. Day by day, ratchet up the number of squeezes until you are able to do about two hundred.

Also visit www.kegel-exercises.com, or look up "Kegel exercise" on an Internet search engine such as Google.com or Dogpile.com.

stresses as butterflies fluttering out of my mind into space, and making positive affirmations to myself.

DO IT FOR LOVE!

It's easy to find time for yourself if you do it in the spirit of love. Get rid of words like "must," "should," and "need"; they bog you down. So never again say:

- I need to fit into that size-eight dress.

- I've got to iron out that wrinkle on my forehead.

- I should do something about those cracks on my heels.

- I must get a treadmill.

Instead, say:

- I'd love to feel lighter on my feet. How about if I make a few soup-and-salad dinners?

- Let's see. I have a few minutes and a few strawberries to spare. Why not treat my face to a quick fruit pack? (Crushed strawberries whisked with cream, applied on the face for a few minutes, and then washed off...yummy!).

- There's nothing like the feel of warm oil, rubbed slowly on my tired feet. Besides what it does for my skin, I love what it does for my nerves!

- A walk in the park with my neighbor/child/dog...won't that be refreshing?

Doesn't this 180-degree attitude rethink feel less like a chore and more like going out to buy a bunch of roses for your sweetheart? That's the spirit!

TOGETHER, THESE CRUMBS OF TIME added up to form a loaf of more than two golden hours in my day. All I had to do was bite into them, savor them, and relish the thought that each morsel of time was going to make me healthier and happier. That's exactly what I did — and the results, I am thrilled to report, have been delicious!

Let me invite you to do the same.

Have a Minute?

GREAT! Let those sixty seconds never slip-slide away again. Make them count: fill them with restorative, refreshing activities. Take a deep breath, drink a glass of water, roll your neck, shrug your shoulders, jog on the spot, eat a banana, share a joke — basically, any little thing that makes you feel good.

On their own, these trivial actions squeezed into one-minute breaks might seem too humble to make a difference. But do some quick addition, and the numbers start to look impressive: Just one minute a day of deep breathing, and in a month you've given yourself thirty precious minutes of more energy, more vitality, more life. All this without making any change in your routine! It really is as easy as it sounds.

Come, let me show you some magical ways in which to maximize a minute.

Inhale Freshness, Exhale Fatigue

BOTH SPIRITUAL GURUS and scientists agree: Good breathing is essential to good living. What exactly do they mean by "good breathing"? This: Don't let breathing be a shallow, in-and-out-of-the-nostrils affair — at least not all day long. If you pause to watch a baby breathe, you'll see that her tummy moves up and down as she inhales and exhales, in an even and easy rhythm. We adults, however, tend to take short, shallow breaths that originate in the upper chest region. This inadequate breathing starves the cells of oxygen and impoverishes the blood. In the long run, it can cause significant health problems such as anxiety, lack of sleep, dizziness, chest pains, disturbed vision, and even hallucinations.

Now look at what happens when you take a minute to fill your lungs with fresh air. Enriched with oxygen, your blood circulates more efficiently, replenishing your tissues and organs with vital nutrients and sweeping toxins out of your system more quickly. Every cell of your being feels more alive, prompting better digestion, improved assimilation of nutrients, and a feeling of overall well-being.

What's more, a breathing break is easy to take. Walk up to an open window or, if you work in a closed environment, simply sit in your chair. Relax your body and feel the warm, moist air as it reaches into and emerges from your lungs. Welcome the stream of fresh air coursing through your body. Picture the stale, toxic air as it exits your body, taking with it your pent-up stress. Feel the tiredness lift from your muscles and the dullness depart your mind.

If you're new to deep breathing, it helps to remember some simple rules:

- While breathing deeply, always sit up straight but not stiffly. An erect posture allows your diaphragm and ribs to move without restriction, improving the quality of your breathing. A simple way to check if you're breathing correctly is to place a hand over your tummy. If it expands and contracts deeply as you inhale and exhale, you're breathing as you should.

- Make sure your clothing is comfortable. Loosen a tight belt or necktie, and unhook your brassiere if need be, to allow your lungs to breathe fully.

• Don't make an effort to breathe; the idea is not to get all tense and uptight. Your neck, shoulders, and back are especially prone to tension, so consciously relax them before you breathe.

Stop, S-t-r-e-t-c-h, Go

IN THE BEST-SELLING BOOK *Chicken Soup for the Writer's Soul,* I came across an inspiring sentence by Howard Fast: "How did I become a writer? That can be answered in one line: the back of my seat to the seat of my chair."[1] To this, let me add a useful tip: Work hard, by all means, but don't subject your muscles to continuous strain from all that sitting.

An aching back and a stiff neck are telling you something urgent: Your muscles are not only fatigued and weak; they are in dire need of some rest and recuperation. Before you know it, that "slight stiffness" can quickly grow into aching arms, shoulders, back, and head. Soon you could even suffer dizzy spells. This happens when there's a logjam in the muscles of your body, slowing down the blood-flow and sapping energy.

Cheer up! It's super-easy to salvage the situation. Whenever you have a minute to spare, stand up and move around. This will instantly get your blood flowing briskly and reduce the strain on your back, neck, and shoulders.

On days when you cannot afford even a few minutes to get up and take a break, try these wonderful in-your-chair exercises:

• Let your hands hang loose, then shake them vigorously for half a minute or so. It's an excellent way to release tension from your fingers. You can do this sitting or standing up. Each time I do it, I visualize myself shaking the stresses loose from my mind, too. It feels supremely comforting.

- Here's a one-minute solution for all that pain in the neck: When you feel your muscles stiffen, press your fingertips gently down your neck and on down to your shoulder blades. You will actually feel the stress slide down with your fingers. Simpler still, roll your head from side to side gently, taking care not to jerk your neck. Very relaxing.

- Sitting comfortably in your chair, slowly roll your shoulders forward, then roll them up towards your ears. Breathing deeply and exhaling fully, hold to a count of five, then lower them gently back into normal position. Repeat five times.

  Now, repeat the stretch in a slightly different way. Instead of rolling your shoulders forward, roll them backwards, and roll them up towards your ears as before. Again, hold for a count of five and then relax. Don't forget to breathe deeply. Take care not to jerk or overstretch your muscles — the idea is to loosen up, not exert yourself. This is a wonderfully simple way to rejuvenate a tired body, especially if you have been working at the computer for a long time.

  I do this regularly and, believe me, it is even more soothing than it sounds. So go on and roll your shoulders at least once a day!

Afraid you'll forget to find time for these simple stretches? Tape a little note above your desk or set a gentle alarm on your computer, reminding you to arch your back, roll your neck, or touch your toes. For even greater benefits, treat yourself to a minute of deep breathing afterward.

Walk Tall

SPEAKING OF MUSCLES, it's impossible not to think about posture. Again, the way you carry yourself is something you can change in an instant — and, happily, the rewards are instantaneous, too.

To begin with, an erect posture is the quickest beauty fix. As you walk down the corridor, straighten your back and hold your head high. How do you feel? A few inches taller, more graceful, and more confident, if I'm not mistaken. For inspiration, remind yourself of Scarlett O'Hara as she swept into the room in *Gone with the Wind*, or the character played by Kate Winslet as she stepped down the staircase in *Titanic*. What made these women such commanding personalities? It was the way they carried themselves: head held high, shoulders squarely thrown back.

There's also another, more important reason for paying attention to your posture: It's good for your health. Correct posture lifts the strain from your muscles and prevents unsightly, potentially harmful humps from forming. Poor posture, on the other hand, cramps your chest and forces you to breathe shallowly. It puts undue pressure on your bones and ligaments, causing your joints to weaken. Poor carriage also compresses your vital organs, forcing digestion to slow down, blood flow to decrease, and the body's self-repair system to work less efficiently — all just because you're in the habit of slouching as you walk and slumping as you sit!

Kick the habit, bit by bit. Here are some simple ways to carry yourself more gracefully:

- If you're sitting at the computer for long periods of time, pause every fifteen minutes to gently rotate your neck from side to side. Roll your shoulders up and down, slowly and without straining them. Do this three to five times each.

- Stand up and rotate your arms in a windmill-like circle, going first clockwise and then counterclockwise. This relaxes the pressure on your neck, shoulders, back, and arms. Do this exercise very gently, to avoid straining a muscle.

- If you've worn high heels to work, take them off as you work at your desk. Pointed heels force your foot and leg muscles to realign themselves unnaturally.

- From time to time, remind yourself to be aware of how your body moves as you walk down the office corridor, through the mall, or in the park. Imagine that you are suspended from the top of your head by a string, and lift your chin to align yourself with it.

- Don't slouch or sit stiffly at your desk. If you're sitting down to watch TV at home, take a moment to adjust your posture: no slumping. If you resolve to sit on the couch only for as long as you can sit up straight, you'll find yourself switching off the TV much sooner than if you lie down and get cozy with a bag of buttered popcorn to boot.

Stroke Your Scalp Happy

JUST LIKE YOUR BODY MUSCLES, your hardworking head needs some relaxation, too. One of the easiest head-helping ideas I know of is to untie my ponytail, then take a brush and run it through my hair. Each time the hairbrush begins its gentle journey down the strands of my hair, it seems to straighten more than knots; it smoothes my jangled nerves and sorts out my thoughts. I guess the real reason that happens is because I've taken the time to stand alone and do something mechanical and nonstrenuous. Try it!

Next time you're feeling confused or hassled at work, retreat to the restroom with a hairbrush. It's a great way to get in touch with your body, using a simple tool and a small amount of time.

Don't think this tip won't work for you if you wear your hair very short. The act of brushing doesn't simply untangle your tresses; it also gives your scalp a mini-massage. The teeth of the comb stimulate hair roots and boost circulation. The gentle tugging action removes scale, dirt, and oils trapped in the follicles and scalp. It also coats the hair with essential sebum, which lubricates, protects, and lends sheen to your mane.

Do invest in the best hairbrush you can find. Your hair will thank you for it, and your mirror will compliment you for it. A brush basic: Natural bristles are best. To find the right brush for your hair, borrow a hair-care book from the library or surf the Internet for tips on the right size and shape for your style. Remember: A good-quality brush will last years and years if you clean it regularly with a gentle shampoo. Hairdressers caution against using harsh products such as vinegar, ammonia, or bleach on your brush; these can cause irreparable damage to the bristles.

Tuck a small brush or comb in your purse. If you forget, smooth out tangles using your fingers; they make the gentlest comb in the world. This works especially well if you have curly hair and cannot run a brush through your hair without making loose curls frizzy.

Freshen up Your Breath

WHILE YOU'RE IN THE RESTROOM, pep up your mouth and mood with a rinse or a toothbrushing; even a quick one is incredibly refreshing. Out go the bacteria, and in comes confidence. With your mouth feeling fresh, you no longer hesitate to smile at people and get close to them. That, in turn, makes you feel good about yourself.

If you can't squeeze in enough time for even a short brushing, just treat your mouth to a clean-water rinse several times a day.

Dentists say that swishing your mouth vigorously with water is an excellent way to flush out bacteria. Remember to rinse your mouth every time you visit the restroom, after every cup of coffee or tea, and after a sweet treat so that bacteria don't have time to react with the acids in sugar, causing cavities and bad breath.

The ancient medical texts of India recommend an interesting way to get your mouth clean and your eyes sparkling at the same time. It's as easy as 1-2-3:

1. Fill your mouth with water.

2. Keeping the water inside your cheeks, gently splash cool water over your eyes five to ten times.

3. Empty the water from your mouth and pat your eyes dry.

In addition to cleaning out your mouth, this is said to improve eyesight and refresh the eyes. If you wear eye makeup during the day, you can try this before leaving for work in the morning and after you return home in the evening.

To keep your breath naturally fresh, munch on carrots, apples, celery sticks, or a sprig of mint. As a bonus, chewing them will exercise your jaws and give you vital nutrients.

Also, keep a travel-sized kit in your purse, containing these items:

• A small toothbrush

• Natural, sugar-free toothpaste

• Nonalcoholic mouthwash

• A stainless-steel tongue-scraper (to tease bacteria out of their favorite hiding place: the furry back of your tongue)

Use this mini mouth-care kit whenever you're feeling dull or low on confidence.

Irrigate Your Skin

CAN YOU REALLY HOPE to care for your skin during those forty frenzied hours of work between Monday and Friday? Absolutely. What does it take? Just one moisturizing minute — a minute during which you hydrate your skin from the inside by treating it to the world's healthiest drink: plain mineral water.

Just three such minutes each day will add up to fifteen minutes in a week and one full hour in a month: sixty glasses of healing water coursing through your system, sweeping away accumulated toxins, and replenishing your cells and tissues.

This, of course, means you should have water available to you during the day. Easy! This coming weekend, stock up on a month-long supply of mineral water and carry a bottle to work every morning (or, space permitting, stock them in the office fridge). In addition to drinking the water, you can also fill a spray bottle with mineral water and spritz it on your face from time to time.

If you stay at home, keep your day's quota of water in an attractive jug, or in your favorite sports bottle, and put it on your dining table. To add allure, float some slices of lemon or cucumber in the water. Whenever you pass by, pour yourself some water in a lovely glass. Sip it slowly with a straw so that you can enjoy it like a soft drink. Really refreshing!

Try to drink your water at room temperature, as iced water can damage the delicate lining of your stomach and slow your metabolic activity.

A variation: Buy the best organic rosewater you can get and squirt it on your face (with your eyes closed) a few times a day. It will wake up more than your skin; all of your five senses will come alive.

You can buy rosewater in a natural food store, but it is more fun — and quite easy — to make it at home.

ROSEWATER

2 cups of fresh rose petals (from your backyard or a natural food store)
1 quart of distilled water

Soak the petals in water for twenty-four hours in a sunny window. Strain the petals out, then use the liquid as desired. A quicker method is to gently heat the petals in the water until almost boiling. Let cool, then strain.

Fill a spray bottle with rosewater and give yourself a rejuvenating spritz a few times during the day. It takes just a few seconds, and look what you get in return: dew-fresh, youthful skin!

Here's another idea to rejuvenate your skin: On evenings when you have a few hours to spare, plan a water-rich vegetable-and-fruit feast for the next day. Visit the supermarket to buy fresh celery, papaya, cucumber, and melons. Slice and pack them in the fridge to take along to work or, if you're staying at home, call up a friend to enjoy them with you.

Revitalize Your Eyes

RIGHT NOW, as you read this, your eyes are hard at work. How long have they been awake and active? Would they like a brief rest? Unless you've just awakened from a nap, I'm sure your answer is "yes!"

Go ahead: Close your eyes. Cup your palms over your eyes and feel the relief flood through your eye muscles and, slowly, through your entire body. "Palming" or "cupping" your eyes a few times a day calms and deepens your breathing, refreshes your mind and body, and gives you a mini-vacation in the comfort of your chair.

Even simpler: Blink. There's more to blinking than meets the eye. The simple action of closing your eyelids replenishes three kinds of fluids in your eyes: tears, oil, and mucus. All of these flush out tiny dust particles, filter out foreign bodies, and coat the eye with essential moisture. Especially when you're engaged in an attention-intensive activity such as sewing, watching a thriller, or working at the computer, do remember to blink. Experts say that a healthy adult eye should open and close about fifteen times a minute. Time your blinks; it might help you decide whether your eyes are under undue strain.

The next tip I'm about to share with you makes me want to close my eyes in pleasure just thinking about it. Imagine that you have just arrived home after being stuck in a long traffic jam. Your eyes are burning from the smog and strain. Obviously, you would love some instant relief. No problem! Pull out a few sterilized cotton balls from your drawer and dampen them with rosewater. Now sink back in an easy chair, close your eyes, and press the cotton gently on your eyelids for a few minutes. Bliss! You can also freeze rose water in an ice tray, wrap the cubes in a clean muslin

INSPIRING QUOTES ABOUT THE HUMAN BODY

If anything is sacred, the human body is sacred.

— Walt Whitman

Every day I am aware of the flow and constant change; perhaps I am at the edge of discovering what more our bodies might be able to teach about the spirit of life . . .

— Ruth Bernhard

The body says what words cannot.

— Martha Graham

Take care of your body with steadfast fidelity. The soul must see through these eyes alone, and if they are dim, the whole world is clouded.

— Johann Wolfgang von Goethe

Water, air, and cleanness are the chief articles in my pharmacy.

— Napoleon Bonaparte

cloth, and place the cloth over your closed eyes. These rosewater ice cubes make a fragrant addition to a glass of drinking water, too.

If you lack the energy for even this simple rosewater treatment, just splash your eyes gently with cold water a few times and dab them dry with a soft towel. You'll feel the stress melt away.

Wouldn't it be great if your eyes could endure that long traffic jam and still feel fresh enough to watch a ninety-minute movie? Well, there's a delicious way to make that possible. All you have to do is eat. Snack on almonds, raisins, papaya, or other sweet, juicy fruits (apples and pears, in particular). Healers in India have prescribed these foods for centuries to nourish the eyes. If you know of something nicer than munching a handful of plump, moist raisins and knowing that you're doing your eyes a favor, do let me know!

Liven up Your Senses with Scent

HAVE YOU EVER NOTICED how a bunch of fresh flowers on the table makes you want to do feel-good things — like cozy up with a book or call a friend over? There's a powerful reason for it. A flower is the very essence of a plant. So, when you take pleasure in its color, texture, and scent, you connect with that which is purest and most healing in nature. Wouldn't you be grateful to have such a life-sweetening sight and scent surround you when you need it most: at work, during your commute, or in the evening after a long day? Good news! You can enjoy fragrance all day long, without splurging on time or money. Some quick and refreshing ideas:

• Do you have a flower vase or two? If you spend most of your time in an office, buy a slim vase that will look good on your desk without taking up too much space.

(If space is really tight, a penholder could do double duty.) Now start keeping a lookout for bouquet bargains in the supermarket, and indulge in them occasionally. For intense fragrance, choose jasmine, hostas, and gardenias. If you enjoy blossoms with a delicate perfume, bring home narcissus, hyacinth, crocuses, or roses. With proper care, your bouquet should last you at least a week, if not more. As soon as you arrive home with your bunch of beauties, tuck them in an attractive vase with fresh water and some preservative powder that usually comes with the bouquet. Next morning, pull out a flower or two from the vase, wrap it in tissue, and carry it to work, where your office vase awaits them. If you're at home, divide the flowers in your bouquet into smaller bunches and tuck them in various places around your house: in the bath, in the kitchen, in your bedroom. Simpler still, if you have a flowerbed in your backyard, treat yourself to a blossom every day!

• So what if you live in a high-rise apartment, have no patience for gardening, or can never remember to look at the fresh-flower aisle? Pick a pleasing scent off your bathroom shelf. Dab a cotton ball with your favorite fragrance and tuck it into your blouse; you'll smell good and feel inspired all day long.

• A variation on the same theme: Douse a natural sponge or clean handkerchief with an essential oil that makes you feel good and tuck it into your bag. Choose oils such as orange, pine, and peppermint to wake up the senses, and select from among geranium, rosemary, and jasmine for relief from anxiety. For an instant

pick-me-up or calm-me-down, mist the sponge or
hanky with water and dab it on your wrists and neck;
the body heat that emanates from these areas will acti-
vate the scents and make them linger longer.

• Fragrant waters have a way of waking up the skin while
simultaneously soothing the soul. I find that the essence
of rose, in particular, is tremendously healing on a hard
day. Buy a good-quality, organic rosewater or lavender
water from a natural health store (or make your own,
using the recipe in this chapter) and spritz it on your
face and neck before applying moisturizer to your skin
(taking care to keep your eyes closed as you spray). A
reminder: After you open a bottle of floral mist, you
should always refrigerate it.

• Here's a terrific way to create your own cologne in
less than a minute: fill an eight-ounce spray bottle
with mineral water and add two drops of your favorite
essential oil. Try lemon or peppermint for a burst of
energy, or lavender or ylang-ylang for a calming effect.
Keep it refrigerated, and spray this hydrating fragrance
on your face and arms for an instant lift whenever you
feel dull. Essential oils can be very potent, so always
check to see if the oil you want to use is safe to inhale
or ingest. It's always advisable to test a portion of the
solution on a small patch of skin to be sure it doesn't
bother you.

In these simple ways, you can fill your life with fragrance.
All the tips I've shared with you are easy and quick, but they're
guaranteed to lift your spirits, boost creativity, and revive happy
memories.

Look, There Goes a Minute!

SEE HOW BEAUTIFULLY you can harvest the humble minute?

The trick is to tease these scraps of time out of their hiding places, say "I spy," and make them your own. So let me show you more nooks and crannies where those precious me-moments hide, waiting for you to discover them.

Basically, you could be feeling time-strapped for two reasons: Either you're spending too much time on activities that are wasteful or unproductive, or you're not spending enough time on the things that really need your attention.

First, take a look at some potential time-wasters in your day:

Surfing the Internet

THERE'S A JOKE GOING AROUND that says, "Five signs that you're a Net nerd: You spend Friday nights with your computer; you've never actually met many of your friends; in an emergency, your first instinct is to e-mail 911; you tell someone your name and end it with 'dot com'; your dog has his own homepage." Funny, yes, but only to an extent. For some of us, the Internet can grow into an addiction that threatens to overshadow other, more important things in our lives. Well, it'll only become worse with time. Unhook yourself from the World Wide Web and set aside a fixed quota of time for surfing. Stick a "Log Off" reminder on a wall that faces you in the computer room. Be sure to change the reminder now and then so that it doesn't become an item you don't notice any longer. Use the time you thus save to give yourself a massage, do a yoga exercise, go for a walk, or dish up something healthy for dinner.

Shopping for Groceries

MOST OF US HAVE A TYPICAL grocery-shopping pattern. Think about yours. Do you enter the supermarket without a clue as to what you'll buy? Worse, do you enter the store famished, wheeling your cart urgently toward the frozen-desserts aisle? What are your favorite aisles, and how much time do you spend scouring them? If your answers reveal a preference for empty, calorie-laden foods such as instant dinners, glazed doughnuts, sweet rolls, candy bars, chips, and breaded snacks, it's time to take stock of your food-shopping habits. The next time you go to the supermarket, enter with a well-thought-out list of healthy food items. Float past those calorie aisles, and invest your time and money in fresh produce, whole grains, and organic juice instead. You'll come back with a cartload of revitalizing nutrients, guaranteed to add years to your life.

Eating Dinner

YES, YOU SHOULD DEFINITELY TAKE TIME to savor your food, so I'm not suggesting that you wolf down your meal. But where you can save time is by avoiding that second helping. Say a firm "no" to another serving of pasta or pie; it's nothing but an additional strain on your stomach and a drain on your time. Instead, take time to chew what's on your plate thoroughly and unhurriedly. This not only allows you to taste every morsel, but also makes it easier for your digestive system to process the meal.

Making Dessert

ALL THAT WHIPPING, folding, and kneading is certainly worth the effort as far as taste is concerned, but wouldn't it be great if you could add nutrition to your desserts while shaving off time? I've got just the idea for you. The next time you make a sweet treat, play with the recipe. To begin with, halve the amount you're going to make:

Reduce those double-layer and double-crust cakes and pies to single layers; they taste just as good, but they have fewer calories. Next, cut down the amount of butter and sugar you use, and increase the quantity of nuts and fruit. Take apple crumble, for instance. If the recipe calls for half a cup of butter, use only one-fourth cup. One cup of sugar? No way. Use only one-fourth cup, enhancing the sweet taste by adding a handful of plump, moist raisins or a spoonful of honey. The results will be very satisfying if you take care to use good-quality, fresh, organic ingredients. Not only will dessert be done more quickly; you'll have all the pleasure, with fewer calories.

SEE? ISN'T IT EASY and exciting to make the same old activities both healthier and less time-consuming?

On the other side of the coin, there are things we tend to rush — but should really spend a few extra minutes on. These activities include:

Moisturizing Your Skin

DOES YOUR MOISTURIZING ROUTINE go something like this: turn cap, squeeze cream, slather it on face and neck, and close cap? Hey! Slow down. That one minute of cream-dabbing before going to bed or while getting ready for work is your chance to give your skin get some much-deserved attention. Let the languid rhythm of your fingers work its way on your neck and shoulders, behind your ears, up your legs. This mini-massage will remove the dead cells from your face, waking it up and making it glow. Your skin will love the feel of your fingertips, relaxing tense muscles and making you feel good about doing something self-nurturing.

Drying Yourself after a Bath

FOR MANY OF US, a morning shower is a rushed affair, and that is understandable. But wait: However harried you might be, you can still squeeze in some healing moments at this time. The trick is to slow down after you've turned off the faucet and picked up the towel. Look at your towel with a fresh sense of respect! It's a great tool for giving you quick exfoliation, a circulation boost, and a mini-massage. Scrub your body well, coaxing out moisture and leftover grime from each curve and crevice. Wipe yourself dry in gentle but firm strokes. Make sure you use a large, thirsty towel that feels good against your skin. You will find it, quite literally, a touching experience.

Brushing Your Teeth

IF YOU'RE ALWAYS RUSHING through brushing, now's the time to slow down and give your pearlies some extra attention. Good, thorough brushing should take not less than two minutes. To make sure you're devoting at least that much time to your teeth, keep a radio or music player by your bathroom sink and play a song while you polish your porcelain gems. Continue brushing at least until the song reaches halfway. As a bonus, you'll get a little musical treat.

Brushing should ideally be followed by thorough flossing, which teases out bacteria from the crevices between teeth and prevents disease-causing plaque from forming. If you cannot find the time to floss both morning and evening, do it at least once before bedtime, because your mouth produces less saliva during sleep, making the environment conducive for bacteria to thrive. Again, this vital activity requires thoroughness and patience. Think of all the time (and money) you might have to spend at the dentist's office if you don't pay attention now.

Cooking Dinner

CREATING A MEAL can be a tremendously healing activity. Every evening, you have an opportunity to connect with your food and your family. Why rush it? Instead, turn it into an adventure — at least on days when you're not dog-tired. Making lentil soup tonight? Think beyond the recipe book. Take a quick peek in your pantry for nourishing additions to the broth. A spoonful of healthy nuts or seeds, a sliced tomato, some grated cheese? You'll get more flavor, extra nutrition, and a new recipe! Similarly, if you're dishing up a salad or cooking pasta, get creative and add your own healthy touch to the recipe. Play with freshly grated lemon zest, fresh herbs, goat cheese, flaxseeds, pecans, apples, prunes, and other wholesome ingredients. Let your kitchen be your studio, where you work with an exciting palette of flavors. Your imagination is the only limit to how nutritious and delicious you can make your meal.

Want more such ideas?

Start Your Own Tip Collection

AS ENDLESS AS PEBBLES and shells on a beach, the world is filled with friendly tips that can help you save time and savor life. Start collecting tips, and you'll soon have a precious set of handy, healthful ideas to use on a harried day.

Observe the good habits of family and friends, and emulate the best ones in your life. Here are a few I gleaned from my own favorite people:

- My mom taught me to always have eggs and boiled potatoes on hand; they're the easiest, most versatile foods to put together in a pinch, and they're nourishing, too.

- My neighbor Katie showed me that saying hello to your plants every morning could be the freshest start to your day.

- Another friend taught me an easy yoga exercise called *tadasana*, which I do every morning while waiting for my coffee to brew. To do tadasana, raise your arms above your head, then slowly rise on your toes. Count to five, lower your feet back to the ground, and let your arms relax at the side of your body. Inhale and exhale slowly while doing the exercise. It improves circulation and gives all your muscles a good stretch.

In addition to people you know, listen to those you have never met. *The Woman's Comfort Book* by Jennifer Louden, *Simple Abundance: A Daybook of Comfort and Joy* by Sarah Ban Breathnach, and *Office Spa: Stress Relief for the Working Week* by Darin Zeer are all good books with fabulous ideas. Wake up to their advice, and take them to bed each night. Start collecting their tips, pin them on your office board, stick them on your fridge, jot them down, and follow as many as you can.

Go to your nearest public library and explore the health section. I'll always be grateful to an unknown voice in the corridor of my local library. Two women were talking, and this is what they said:

"I just don't have time to read anymore, what with the children. You know how it is..."

Her friend replied, "Yeah, but you know, I've come up with this excellent solution: I pick up the tiniest books I can find. They're cute, and they are pocket-sized. They fit nicely in your palm, they're easy to browse, and they almost always leave you with one tip that sticks in your mind."

So scan the shelves of your public library for some tiny treasures. I did, and look what I found within five minutes:

1. A pocket guide on how to plan a healthy meal, how to control your portions, and how to tell fat from fit. For example, when you go to a restaurant, look out for clues that signal "fat-laden":

HIGHER FAT	LOWER FAT
Au gratin	Steamed
Breaded	Roasted
Creamed	Au jus, or in its own juice

2. A ready-reckoner on how to buy the freshest products at the supermarket and cook them to perfection. One of the tips I liked: If the fresh vegetables in the aisle look wilted or old, inquire about whether the store has any fresher produce — and don't be shy about asking!

3. A pocket-sized book about carrots, with delicious recipes for iced carrot-and-orange soup; carrot, tofu, and rice casserole with toasted almonds; and brown-sugar carrot pudding. The advantage with this sort of book is that you can flip through it during lunch-break at the office, choose what you'd like to cook for dinner, and shop on your way home for a bunch of bright carrots and any other ingredients you might need.

See what a wealth of revitalizing information you can cull from a handful of pages? Isn't it a fun way to make life zestier? But wait, I have an even better idea — one that is sure to send you to the stationery store in search of an attractive notebook.

Create a Joyful Living Journal

ALL IT TAKES IS PAPER and a pen, and you can start growing your own garden of tips. Set aside one minute a day to write a feel-good note in your new journal: a fun piece of information you heard, thoughts, ideas. Write down how you are feeling at the moment. Or think up revitalizing resolutions such as these: "I'll take a barefoot stroll on the lawn this evening; stop on my way home to buy good-quality honey for apple compote; or soak my feet in a bucket of warm water, trim my nails, then rub in foot cream." Keeping this journal will help you connect with yourself once a day and fill you with anticipation at the thought of the little pleasures that await you after the duties of the day are done.

THOUGHTS FROM HELEN BACKER,
RETIRED ACCOUNTING MANAGER, 73

How to enjoy your body to the fullest:

1. Pamper your body. When I was working, I did little things to make me happy. I would go for a jog before I fixed dinner, or make a martini and sip it slowly in the porch, or play with my cat.

2. A happily employed body is a healthy body! Find something creative to do even if you think you have no talent. Take classes. You would be surprised at what you can do. I currently glass-paint and knit. It is even better when you can paint, do ceramics, or engage in some other creative activity with a couple of friends.

3. Stay active! Go adventuring; do out-of-the-ordinary things even if it scares you a bit. It's hard to describe the thrill of doing something you challenged yourself to do. (For me, this could be running a race or backpacking on a mountain.)

Just like this, page by page, moment by healing moment, you can bless yourself with grace, charm, and enough energy to give away — a joie de vivre that permeates your mind and heart and shows up in the way you walk, talk, look, and perform.

Then, when a colleague asks you to share your secret, by all means do so! Tell her the good news that it is perfectly possible to improve one's health without making drastic changes in one's routine. Who knows, you could turn her life around, too. Share your happy secret with your friends, spouse, and kids. Together, you can all discover the joy of better living, minute by therapeutic minute.

In the following chapters, I'll take you on a healing journey that spans your home, your hearth, and your mind. Together, we'll watch hundreds of refreshing vistas unfold, all while going about the mundane business of life.

Read on!

Chapter Summary and Resources

- You can live more healthfully on your busy schedule by juggling your time just a little. Take a little me-minute here, a few self-care seconds there. Inspire yourself to live more fully with books about comfort. I recommend *Self-Nurture: Learning to Care for Yourself as Effectively as You Care about Everyone Else,* by Alice D. Domar (Viking Press, 1999), and *The Woman's Comfort Book: A Self-Nurturing Guide for Restoring Balance in Your Life,* by Jennifer Louden (Harper, 1992).

- An estimated 90 percent of us are not breathing the right way: deeply, slowly, and calmly. Come on: Inhale more oxygen and energy! Exhale that stress and those stale gases. On the website www.breathing.com, you'll find several useful articles on how to breathe well. Created by breath-trainer Michael Grant White, the site offers workshops, seminars, lectures, and videos on the art of breathing. I'm sure you'll find several other breath-training options on the Internet. Another great idea is to learn meditative breathing. Sign up for a yoga class, which teaches you how to breathe for relaxation. Or enroll in judo, karate, or aikido. Most martial arts classes will train you to breathe more fully.

• The word "posture" means "attitude" for a reason. The way you sit, stand, walk, and lie down not only affects your health, but also reflects your general attitude toward life. Check out www.ergonomics.org for articles and information on better posture. The site also offers a course in posture improvement through the Alexander Technique.

• It takes less than a minute to drink a glass of water, but the benefits are tremendous. Water detoxifies, cleanses, lubricates, and replenishes moisture that is vital to the cells. Quench your thirst for more information with *The Complete Book of Water Healing,* by Dian Dincin Buchman (Instant Improvement Publishers, 1995).

• Aroma is therapy! Flowers and their essences can create a powerful alchemy between you and nature. Happily for us, aromatherapy experts have classified essential oils according to their effects on our emotions. My favorite resource for mining this information is the book *Aveda Rituals,* by Horst Rechelbacher (Henry Holt and Company, 1999).

• Whatever you do for your body, do it with love and not from a sense of duty — just like you would for your sweetheart!

CHAPTER 2

Nourishment

How to Savor the Bounteous Flavors of Health

If women but knew it, health is more apt to be maintained
by what is done by them in the kitchen than by [what] all the
doctors and druggists can do for their families

— RALPH BORSODI

My friend Sylvia has the kind of home that hugs you. Her kitchen is always warm with the scent of fresh food; today it's cinnamon, tomorrow it could be basil and roasted garlic. Baskets of bread, bowls of ripe red apples, and heaps of nuts fill the table. When she opens the fridge for a carton of cream, you glimpse a treasure-trove of color: fresh green parsley, brown eggs, crimson strawberries, bright orange carrots, tall jugs of juice, a pitcher of milk. Sylvia thinks her kitchen could do with more sunshine and less clutter. I think it is one of the brightest, most comforting places in the world.

To me, Sylvia epitomizes *annapoorna*, a Hindi word for "one who nourishes." The ancient healers of India used the word as a synonym for woman herself. "Annapoorna" is a synthesis of *anna* (grain) and *poorna* (fulfilling), and it describes the fullness of Sylvia's life: from errands to children to volunteer work. Not surprisingly, Annapoorna is also the Hindu goddess of nourishment.

There's one other annapoorna I know, and that is my mother. To this day, ask me to describe my mother and I'll grope among words like "gentle," "soft," and "sweet" — but ask me how she smells, and I'll say, with a catch in my throat, "Oh, she smells of lime and curry leaves and a whiff of tender green mango."

Awaken the Annapoorna in You

HAPPILY, you don't have to give up your job, change your priorities, and break your back to become an annapoorna. All it takes is:

- A fresh-as-lemons zest for living a more wholesome, nourishing life,
- A few ounces of your time, and
- Some generous scoops of creativity.

Ready with these basics? Then let's go! I'll show you how to be the goddess of nurturing in easy, exciting ways.

Begin with Your Shopping Basket

LET'S SAY THAT, starting today, you resolve to eat a balanced diet. How would you proceed? By looking at a chart? If so, I'm afraid one look at those listings of daily dietary requirements — B1, thiamine, B2, riboflavin, pantothenic acid, sodium, potassium, cobalt, selenium, molybdenum, tryptophan, methionine, et cetera — would make you feel overwhelmed and defeated even before you begin.

But this is what one of my favorite authors, Gayelord Hauser, has to say about such lists: "I refuse to reduce the joy of good eating to fine measurements. It discourages the busy person, whose table is not set with a balance scale along with a fork and knife."

I totally agree.

There is a better way to eat a balanced diet than fussing over all those minerals and vitamins. It is this: Step by simple step, master the art of healthy shopping.

At this point, are you saying, "Ah! Been there, read that. Old habits die hard, and no amount of advice can change the way I've been eating for years"? If so, please wait! I promise I'm not asking you to make any dramatic changes or drastic resolutions. I know only too well that they won't last; they don't work. What I'm inviting you to do is something incredibly simple.

Try this: Next time you go grocery shopping, catch yourself "awares" as you stand in front of the ice-cream or candy or cake-mix aisle. That is, become present in that crucial decision-making moment. Imagine that you are there now, planted in front of the ice-cream aisle, poised to make a delicious decision: "Almond Praline" or "Butter Pecan"? "Chocolate-Chip Cookie Dough" or "Rocky Road"?

Now is the time! Close your eyes just for a moment and ask yourself this vital question: "When was the last time I (and my family members) ate something this calorie-rich and heavy?" If the answer is "three weeks or many moons ago," go ahead and indulge. But if it is "three hours ago" or "yesterday," summon up your willpower and push your cart just a few steps ahead so that you are now facing the "low-fat ice-creams" and "sorbet" section. Better still, bypass this aisle and move toward the fresh-fruit zone.

Next, take a look at those enticing packets of instant mashed potatoes. "Fluffy!" "Extra Creamy!" they scream, seducing you with richly colored pictures of melted cheese and herb toppings. Halt a moment before you pop a packet in your cart. Turn the package over and glance at the list of ingredients. Does it run something like this: potato flakes (color and flavor protected with sodium bisulfite, citric acid, and BHA), monoglycerides, sodium acidpyrophosphate? If so, ask yourself: Does your stomach really need all those sulfites and glycerides? Should you be paying for something that might harm you? The answer should help you propel your cart toward the fresh-produce aisle for a handful of potatoes, whose dull brown skins promise nothing, but deliver a great deal of nutrition and flavor.

Now, even if you're too rushed to do anything but microwave your fresh potato, you'll have the satisfaction of knowing that you said "no" to chemicals you don't need. Besides, no brand of packaged potatoes can pack as much flavor and texture as the real thing.

After having tried — and failed at — many other approaches, I've found this stop-and-think method to be the most practical and doable. Of course, it helps tremendously that for every fattening, empty food, there is a healthy, tasty alternative today.

Here are some healthy choices you can make, just by changing the direction of your shopping cart:

REJECT	SELECT
Soda	Nonsynthetic fruit juice
Cream-sandwich cookies	Graham crackers
Frosted cereal	Muesli or oatmeal
Chocolate syrup	Fruit spread or fresh fruit
Pound-cake mix	Whole-wheat pancake mix
Chocolate doughnuts	Bran muffins/ angel food cake
Canned fruit in heavy syrup	Canned fruit in light syrup, or fresh fruit
Three-cheese pasta	Herb-and-garlic pasta or whole-wheat spaghetti
Roasted, salted nuts	Raw, unsalted nuts

Congratulate yourself for every harmful ingredient you discard and every healthful one you buy. You've chosen to be fit instead of fat, healthy instead of heavy. Soon enough, your body will thank you and reward you with extra energy, glowing skin, and more stamina. Not only that, but the health of your whole family will blossom. All this, just because you've begun taking a few seconds in your day to pause and think.

With so much good food to choose from, putting together three healthful meals a day should be a breeze, right? Aha! I know your answer to that: Where's the time? But once again, let me assure you that your answer can change — and quite easily, too. Once again, the trick is to be patient and to bring on the changes bite by delicious bite.

Let's begin with the most important meal of the day.

Take a Fresh Look at Breakfast

WHO CAN DENY that the day goes much better when you've eaten a fortifying meal in the morning? Then what's the problem? Why do we often make do with coffee and toast or, worse, nothing at all? The reason — or, more accurately, the excuse — is familiar: lack of time.

Rejoice! You can wake up to a healthy breakfast no matter how fast you're racing. Here are some easy tips to get you started:

- Wake up fifteen minutes earlier than usual to get a head start on your day. A wise man said, "Lose an hour in the morning, and you will be hunting for it all day." As a corollary, I would say, "Gain a minute in the morning, and you will reap the benefits all day."

- If you simply cannot open your eyes early, prepare for breakfast the night before. An example: Keep some diced fruit (such as strawberries, peaches, mango, and banana) in the blender, and refrigerate or freeze the blender jar overnight. In the morning, add a cup of yogurt or skimmed milk to the fruit, and blend for a minute. You've got an instant vitamin-and-mineral-rich smoothie! Or you can wrap leftover veggies, rice, or salad in a tortilla in the evening and refrigerate it until morning.

• If you really must rush, there are dozens of foods that you can "grab-and-go." Choose from among whole-grain bagels, muffins, bread with peanut butter or fruit spread, raisins, fruit (fresh, canned, or diced from your supermarket's salad bar), yogurt, graham crackers, low-fat cottage cheese, fig bars, hard-boiled eggs, rice cakes, low-sodium vegetable juice, and fruit juice. In a pinch, I sometimes smear a *chapati* (see recipe under Bread and

ONE WORD THAT CAN HELP YOU
EAT MORE HEALTHFULLY

No, that word is not "willpower" or "dieting." It is, quite simply, "frugality." I have living proof of the power of frugality.

Far away from the continent of America, tucked high up in the remote hills of northwestern Pakistan, there lives a tribe of men and women who enjoy vigorous health at the ripe young age of 100 — and many of them live to be nearly 120. All of these people, known as the Hunzas, have perfect 20–20 vision, excellent skin texture, strong teeth, and no trace of coronary artery disease, high blood pressure, or elevated cholesterol levels.

What is their secret?

They eat frugally, consuming at least 1,000 calories less than the average American every day.

Better, page 38) with peanut butter, wrap it around a banana, and enjoy it on my way to work.

On days when you're lucky enough to have a little more time for breakfast, don't settle for the usual pancake-and-eggs routine. Apart from time constraints, one major reason we neglect breakfast is that it is often an unexciting déjà vu experience. Donna Leahy, author of a delicious book called *Morning Glories,* echoes this sentiment. She declares that "most breakfasts are boring,"[1] and shares her recipes for mouthwatering breads, soufflés, cocktails, and even breakfast soups.

Beyond a point, doughnuts, oatmeal, orange juice, and even your favorite blueberry pancakes can get predictable and unappetizing. Solution: Wake up those bored taste buds. Think out of the cereal box!

INSTEAD OF	TRY
Hash browns	Spicy potatoes (see recipe, page 56), or roasted beets laid over toast or slid inside pita bread, or sweet potatoes cooked slowly in olive oil, with a hint of rosemary and garlic added at the last moment
Regular pancakes	Buckwheat, rice flour, or blue cornmeal pancakes
Waffles with maple syrup	Waffles topped with honey, nuts, chopped fruit, raisins, or wheat germ

Danish or doughnut	Fruit drizzled with honey
Cream cheese	Cottage cheese or ricotta cheese on toast or inside bagels — or, for a delicious nondairy alternative, try hummus or avocado on toast or on a bagel
Store-bought flavored yogurt	Fresh homemade plain yogurt (see recipe under A Cupful of Calcium, below) blended with sliced fruit
Orange juice	A whole orange; freshly squeezed orange juice; pineapple, carrot, or apple juice; a luscious smoothie or cocktail
Your second cup of coffee	Mint- or lemon-flavored green tea

Get adventurous! Try these unusual recipes for a va-va-vroom morning:

A CUPFUL OF CALCIUM

Silken, creamy top, and luscious fruit on the bottom — nothing quite compares to store-bought yogurt, right? Unless you make your own yogurt at home. Once you discover that fresh homemade taste, I'm sure you'll never buy a carton of yogurt again. Health-wise, too, it's a good idea; the longer yogurt sits on store shelves, the more friendly bacteria it loses. Besides, store-bought yogurt can be sour. Making yogurt at home is a breeze — and less expensive.

Boil four cups of milk in a pan. Let it cool for a bit, until it feels just warm to the touch. (If you live in a warm place, let the milk cool down completely.) Now pour the milk into a medium-size bowl, and stir in one tablespoon of yogurt until it is completely blended with the milk. Cover the bowl, and let it rest in a warm place overnight or for a few hours (yogurt takes longer to set if you live in a cooler region). To check if the yogurt is done, shake the bowl gently after a few hours. If the liquid is firm and doesn't shake like jelly, your yogurt is ready. Whisk it lightly and stir in some freshly chopped bananas or apples, or a few grapes. Add a bit of honey if you like. For a new flavor, whisk the yogurt in the blender with sea salt, black pepper, and roasted cumin seeds. Or try your own creative ideas; a friend of mine occasionally adds chocolate chips to the yogurt for fun. Since this yogurt is fresh, save one table-spoon of "seed" yogurt from it to make your next batch. Keep this starter refrigerated until you are ready to make more yogurt. For best results, use the starter within two days; after then, it starts to lose its freshness.

A STEW-PENDOUS START

Start your morning with a stewed apple! One medium-sized apple is a treasure-house of vitamins, minerals, and fiber. While apples are delicious simply munched raw, the tradi-tional healers of India recommend cooking them lightly for easier digestion. This recipe comes to you courtesy of my friend Vaidya Ramakant Mishra, an eminent Ayurvedic scholar and physician based in America. (Ayurveda is a system of healing that originated in India more than 5000 years ago. For more information, please see my book *Essential Ayurveda*.)

Soak a tablespoon of raisins overnight. In the morning, peel and make small cubes of one organic apple. Place the apples, raisins, and one clove in a small pan with about one cup of water. When the water boils, reduce the heat to a simmer and cook until the fruit is tender. Discard the clove and enjoy your warm, nutritious apple-raisin stew.

A Handful of Almonds

Shell the almonds and soak them overnight in a cup of water. (You can also buy a bag of pre-shelled almonds to make things easier). Peel the brown skins off them in the morning (they'll slide off easily), and munch them just like that. Or you can toss them into a blender with milk or yogurt for an energizing start to your day. Packed with vitamins, almonds have been credited with improving eyesight and memory.

Bread — and Better!

Have you ever eaten a chapati? Made from whole-wheat flour, a chapati is a delicious, nutritious disk-shaped bread. In India, millions of people eat them for breakfast. You can enjoy chapatis in hundreds of ways: Smear them with herbed butter, or cream cheese, or peanut butter; enjoy them with roasted potatoes and yogurt; fill them with scrambled eggs and roll them up into burritos.

To make chapatis, knead one cup of whole-wheat flour with just enough water to make a soft, smooth dough. Cover and allow the dough to rest for a few minutes. Heat a shallow cast-iron griddle on the stove on maximum heat. Meanwhile, divide the dough into six equal balls, and roll each into a thin circle. (At this point, you can freeze the rolled-out circles in a zip-lock bag until ready to cook). One by one, cook the circles of dough on the hot griddle, turning them over from time to time, until the chapatis puff up and are flecked with brown spots. You will need to fine-tune the heat while cooking the chapatis; generally, it needs to be lowered slightly. Because stove temperatures vary, you will arrive at the right temperature for your chapatis with a little practice. If you're new to chapati-making, try your first batch on a relaxed weekend.

SANDWICH-CRAFT

Take three boiled potatoes and slice them thin or mash them. Now heat two teaspoons of olive oil in a pan on medium heat, and throw in some cumin or oregano seeds (1/4 teaspoon), salt (to taste), mango powder (1/2 teaspoon; it's called *amchoor*, and you'll find it in Indian grocery stores, or you can substitute a teaspoon of lemon juice for it), and spice up the proceedings with just a dash of cayenne pepper (1/4 teaspoon). When the spices start sizzling in the pan, add the potatoes and stir-fry for a few minutes until the potatoes are flecked with gold. Add a few finely chopped cilantro leaves. Next, spoon the potatoes between slices of whole-wheat bread, or insert them in English muffins or bagels. This recipe may sound lengthy, but it takes only a few minutes to make — if you keep boiled potatoes handy in the fridge (they usually keep well for at least three to four days).

SUNSHINE IN A GLASS

Two carrots, two tomatoes, one beet. Together, they make nutritional magic in a juicer. Spike this wake-me-up juice with a piece of ginger, a sprig of mint, or a twist of lime. Power it with lightly roasted sesame seeds, wheat grass, or spirulina.

Here are some more juices and smoothies for a sprightly morning:

- 1 pitted nectarine + 1 cup orange juice + 1/2 cup strawberries + crushed ice (if using fresh fruit)

- 1 chopped apple + 3 pitted dates + 2 cups water + cinnamon to taste

- 1 sliced banana + 1 small bowl of pineapple chunks + 1 cup orange juice + 1/2 cup crushed ice (if using fresh fruit)

- 1 cup sliced fresh or frozen unsweetened peaches + 1/2 cup fresh or frozen raspberries + 1 cup nonfat peach yogurt + 1/2 cup peach nectar + a few ice cubes (if using fresh fruit)

For all of these, the procedure is the same: Process in a blender until smooth, then pour into a glass or travel mug. For best result, peel, cut, and freeze your fruit ahead of time. You will not need to add any ice to make your smoothies if you do this, and they will blend up rich and thick.

BREAKFAST IS JUST the first course in your day, but it can be the beginning of a dramatic change in the way you eat, look, and feel. Breakfast is easy to work off; it boosts your mood; and it helps you perform at peak energy levels. But remember, a "good" breakfast does not mean a heavy one. Eat just enough in the morning to feel energetic, not stuffed. Then, come noon, you can enjoy a hearty, wholesome lunch.

Ooh La Lunch!

I HAVE SOME HAPPY ADVICE for all of you who love to eat, regardless of your weight: Eat lunch queen-size! The logic is simple: Eating a healthful, high-octane lunch recharges you for an afternoon of hard work. But miss lunch or eat a paltry one, and you're guaranteed to overeat later in the day. Result: You're also guaranteed to put on weight, because digestive energy slows down in the evening and the excess food only piles up as layers of fat tissue.

So go ahead and enjoy an afternoon fiesta. Take your brown bag from boring to bustling. Think beyond cheesy sandwiches and greasy burgers. Here are some interesting ideas to get you thinking afresh:

Healthy makeovers for your afternoon meal:

INSTEAD OF	TRY
White-flour bread	Pumpernickel, rye, or whole-wheat bread
Iceberg lettuce	Green-leaf, red-leaf, or romaine lettuce; spinach; arugula
Bologna	Hummus

Salami or pastrami	Hard-boiled eggs in pita bread
Regular mayo	Low-fat mayo — better, no mayo!
Regular cheese	Lite cheese
Potato chips	Pretzels, reduced-fat crackers, Triscuits with cheese
Cupcake	Bran muffin
Soda or "fruit" drinks	100% fruit or vegetable juice
Greasy fast-food burgers	Veggie burgers
Cup of noodles	Hearty lentil soup

Instead of using mayo or cheese, you can make yogurt cheese at home. Simply drain out the water from low-fat yogurt by leaving it overnight in a strainer lined with muslin cloth. Seasoned with dill, sea salt, and crushed black pepper, this yogurt makes a creamy spread or dip.

A word about quality: it pays to spend money on good produce! I know that natural, organic foods can be expensive. If you cannot regularly shop at a natural food store, try shopping there every other weekend for your coming week's supplies, or see if you can cut costs elsewhere so that you can spend more on good-quality food. One way of cutting costs is

FIVE WONDERFUL WAYS TO CONNECT WITH YOUR FOOD

1. Churn buttermilk
2. Grind your own grain
3. Make peanut butter or fruity yogurt at home
4. Cook fresh bread
5. Grill your vegetables

to buy whole foods instead of prepared ones, and you will save enough to cover the costs of switching to organic produce. If elaborate grocery shopping seems too time-consuming, try ordering your supplies through catalogs or on the Internet. (Look for resources in the Chapter Summary and Resources section at the end of this chapter.)

How to Pack Your (Brown) Bag

USE SATURDAYS to relax and rejuvenate. On Sundays, spend some time preparing for your five days of lunch ahead. Some ideas:

- Make a big batch of banana bread or muffins to last you the whole week.

- If you're cooking noodles, pasta, rice, or soup for Sunday dinner, double the amount so you can carry some for lunch the next few days.

- Hard-boil several eggs and potatoes, then keep them in the fridge so you can use them to dish up sandwiches and salads during the week.

- Buy fresh vegetables, then chop and pack them in plastic containers that you can store in the fridge and conveniently carry to work. (I like to chop vegetables while watching television; it doesn't seem like such a chore that way.)

- Invest in precut vegetables if you don't find time to buy and chop them; the nutrition you'll get from them is worth every bit of expense.

- Freeze fruit for a tote-along treat. I enjoy frozen grapes, and so can you. Simply wash seedless grapes and freeze them in zip-lock bags. Carry them to work, and by noon they'll be nice and crunchy. Plus, you'll find that they taste even sweeter this way. Similarly, you can freeze skinned, chopped bananas to whip up smoothies.

Even if Sunday went by in the blink of an eye and you couldn't chop or cook anything ahead, don't give up! Whenever you go grocery shopping, look for prepackaged lunch items of the healthy kind. You can pick from among different varieties of breads and bagels, muffins, oranges, bananas, grapes, nuts, chick-peas, cottage cheese, crackers, juicy carrots, organic yogurt, cartons of organic juice, and condiments such as honey, sun-dried tomato paste, and horseradish. The choices are exciting, so be adventurous — and your "brown" bag will soon crackle with color, flavor, and energy!

Once you've stocked up on a variety of items to last you the whole week, combine them to give you a balance of nutrition and flavors — a little bit each of protein, carbohydrates, and vitamins, salty, sour, and sweet flavors. Let your appetite tell you what quantities are right for your queen-sized meal.

Here are some combinations that I find easy and enjoyable:

- yogurt + pita bread + banana + honey
- apple + peanut butter + bagel + juice
- carrots + hummus + pumpernickel bread + grapes
- salad + boiled egg + whole-wheat bread + raisins
- cottage cheese + wheat-bran muffin + orange or papaya

Take time to think up your own combinations; it's enjoyable and highly rewarding. Even better, involve your friends, family, and colleagues in this fun exercise.

Now I can almost hear you protest, "But this isn't how my body is conditioned to eat! For years now, dinner has been my main meal of the day because that's when I have time to dish up a real meal." But believe me: Rethinking the quantity and quality of your dinner could be your key to a lifetime of healthy eating.

The Case for Dining Lightly

A HEAVY DINNER, eaten late in the evening, can linger in the stomach for up to six hours. The feeling of fullness interferes with the quality of your sleep, making you toss and turn throughout the night. No wonder, then, that when you wake up in the morning you feel you can do with just juice and coffee.

Now imagine treating yourself to a healthful, early dinner. Great decision! To begin with, you'll sleep better. No gas, no bloating, no heartburn, no piling up of pounds overnight. And when you wake up in the morning, you'll welcome that hearty whole-wheat bagel and those fluffy eggs. Congratulations! You're now on your way to a lifetime of rhythmic eating.

If you've been eating big dinners for as long as you can remember, it may take some time for you to adjust to the reduction in quantity. Don't give up in frustration. During the first few days or weeks of your transition, save some soup or salad from your dinner; if you're famished later in the evening, you can have that set-aside food when the hunger pang hits. I find a spoonful of honey satisfying, too.

Here are some other light-snack options for a late-night attack of the munchies:

- celery sticks dipped in cream cheese
- carrot sticks dipped in light sour cream with dill

- apple or pear slices spread with a thin layer of peanut butter and some wheat germ
- half a bowl of fresh berries or pineapple chunks with low-fat cottage cheese
- a low-fat fruit cereal bar with a drizzle of honey
- two rice cakes topped with a thin layer of melted chocolate
- a sliced apple spread with a quarter-teaspoon of peanut butter over each wedge

Not only are these ideas delicious, but they're also satisfying enough to help you avoid binging on chips and other greasy snacks.

So sit down with your family and write up a new dinner menu. It needn't be paltry and uninspiring — just light. Since evening is the time when you can probably afford to take some time to create a more nourishing meal, do take advantage of that. Play with ingredients, mixing and matching them for more power and punch.

Here are three of my favorite dinner ideas:

KHICHRI

Soak 1 cup each of washed long-grain rice and mung dal (green split lentils) in 4 cups of water for 30 minutes. Then heat a tablespoon of *ghee* (clarified butter — available at most Indian grocery stores or see the sidebar on page 54 for an easy recipe to make it at home) in a pan on medium heat, and add cumin seeds or two pods of clove to it. When the seeds or pods begin to splutter, drain out the soaking water from the dal and rice and put them in the pan with salt to taste, then add 6 cups of water. Cook until the grains are completely tender. For extra flavor and nutrition, you can also add chopped green beans, potatoes, spinach, or cauliflower to the hot ghee before adding the lentils.

QUICCHINI

I love to cook zucchini this way. Cut zucchini into small, thin rounds. Finely chop half an onion and a tomato. Crush a clove of garlic and a small piece of fresh ginger. Heat olive oil in a pan on medium heat, add the crushed garlic and ginger, salt to taste, and add the onion and tomatoes. When the paste is soft, add the zucchini rounds and stir to coat thoroughly. Add $1/2$ cup of water to the vegetables, then cover and cook until done — about 20 minutes. This is delicious with fresh whole-wheat or corn bread.

HERBED BRUSCHETTA

Toast four slices of crusty Italian bread until lightly browned on both sides. Rub the slices with raw halved garlic cloves, and top with pepper and freshly chopped basil leaves. Enjoy warm with corn or tomato soup.

Think One Slice, One Dash, One Pinch

IT'S AMAZING what a simple addition can do for your bowl of soup or your plate of salad. Sample this nutrition information:

- One ounce of roasted soybean nuts packs 10 grams of protein and 5 grams of fiber. Surf www.soyfoods.com for exciting, soy-based recipes.

- One ounce of peanuts roasted without oil endows you with 7 grams of protein. For some delicious, peanut-based recipes, check out www.nationalpeanutboard.com.

- One medium apple charges you with 340 kilojoules of energy. Not only that, it gives you about 73 IU of vita-min A, along with a host of other vitamins and essential amino acids. For irresistible apple-based recipes, drop by www.nyapplecountry.com.

- One wedge or slice of lemon squirted over salad gets you nearly 10 mg of potassium and about 4 mg of vitamin C. You'll find some luscious lemon recipes in the book *Lemon Tree Very Healthy: Zestful Recipes with Just the Right Twist of Lemon* by Sunny Baker (Avery Penguin Putnam, 1995).

- One cup of organic low-fat milk gives you 285 mg of calcium, plus generous amounts of phosphorus, potassium, and vitamin A.

SIGHTS, SOUNDS, AND SMELLS
OF A WARM AND WELCOMING KITCHEN

- Herbs and flowers drying from coat hooks and old racks
- A handsome, worn pine table topped with a milk pitcher and lots of fruit
- Enameled metal and wicker containers
- Herbs growing on the windowsill
- Fresh, whole spices or nuts being roasted
- An assortment of herb-infused oil bottles lined up on a shelf
- A clean, comfortable rug underfoot
- A refrigerator and baskets brimming with fresh organic produce
- Lots of cutting boards and knives in different shapes and sizes
- The smell of a cinnamon-flavored fruit pie baking in the oven

I can almost hear you say, "Just one slice of this and one scoop of that? Sounds doable." It is! To me, this one-scoop-one-slice approach has become a daily adventure, to the extent that I've become something of a master innovator. Even if it's just a simple drink of water, I like to perk it up with rose petals and cardamom, which are known to have soothing properties. A squeeze of lemon is wonderful too; it's a good source of vitamin C and a natural diuretic to help cleanse the system. Besides, adding flavor to your water is fun!

Here are some of my favorite one-ingredient ideas; I am sure they will inspire you to think up your own:

- One tablespoon of freshly grated coconut: Sprinkle it on your salad, soup, or dessert. In addition to lending flavor, coconut is believed by the traditional healers of India to improve hair and skin texture, boost metabolism, promote restful sleep, and nourish the mind. Besides, it's moist and sweet and crunchy!

- One teaspoon of fiber-rich bran: Stir it into yogurt, soup, or fruit juice to pack your snack with extra nutrition.

- One twist of lemon: Squeeze it onto hot lentils, baked potatoes, or salad. Enjoy the tang of citrus and the healing benefits of vitamin C.

- One tablespoon of fresh cottage cheese, or even store-bought ricotta: Crumble it on top of fruit or fresh greens to add texture to your salads, brighten them with its pristine whiteness, and load you with calcium, folate, and phosphorus.

- One tablespoon of olive oil: Stir it in next time you steam veggies — especially in December! We think of fresh steamed vegetables as among the healthiest foods, and rightly so. But did you know that, according to traditional Indian wisdom, eating steamed vegetables in the winter months can actually have a drying influence on the skin? For a healthy, moisturizing platter, use olive oil.

Think up some one-derful ideas of your own. Jot them down and stick them on your fridge. Next time you cook dinner, use the one that appeals to you most.

Dessert Rhapsody

IF DINNER IS DONE, can dessert be far behind? Yes, rejoice! It's time for some sweet talk! Imagine a sweet, melt-in-your-mouth treat that pleases your palate without piling up the pounds. Can it be? Absolutely! Here are ten scrumptious ways to help you enjoy that sweet bite without an ounce of guilt:

1. Let dessert be a spoonful of the best honey you can get. Replete with vital minerals and vitamins, honey satisfies the sweet tooth without adding empty calories.

2. Enjoy sliced fruit and cheese after your meal — very satisfying, and a natural way to freshen the mouth, too. Some ideas: Try sliced green apples with sharp cheddar cheese, fresh blueberries or strawberries with fat-free whipped topping, or almost any fruit with honey.

3. If you absolutely crave a slice of cake once a day, reserve dessert as an after-lunch treat instead of a post-dinner one; your system is geared to take on bigger amounts of food during daytime.

4. Serve puddings in small, shallow bowls; slice cakes and pies thin. A little portion control will go a long way in saving you calories.

5. Train your taste buds to enjoy lightly sweetened desserts. It's easy if you use molasses, maple syrup, spreadable fruit, or fresh fruit purée instead of sugar.

6. Instead of making double-crust pies, use lattice-patterned pastry cuttings to top a pie; you'll cut calories and add visual appeal.

7. Even if you're baking a simple batch of cookies, try to make them more vitamin-and-fiber-rich by adding healthy ingredients, such as dates, raisins, and cranberries. Further, substitute maple syrup, applesauce, blackstrap molasses, or honey for sugar to subtract calories and add flavor to your cookies.

8. Skewer fresh fruit on toothpicks for a good-looking, delicious, healthy dessert. Or, make your own "juicicles." An example: Mash a mango or three peaches, add a cup of orange juice to the fruit, then pour this luscious mixture into an ice tray. Cover with plastic wrap, stick toothpicks in, and you will have a healthy, sorbet-like frozen pop, Invite your kids to make these fruit kabobs and popsicles with you; when they feel involved in preparing dessert, they'll find it delicious, too!

9. A light dessert doesn't have to be an unappetizing one. Garnish it with a few fresh berries, edible flowers, or a sprig of mint, and your simple treat of poached peaches will immediately look more alluring.

10. Add naturally sweet-tasting vegetables such as carrots and peas to your diet; they'll reduce your craving for artificial, sugary desserts.

See what delicious possibilities the world of flavor holds? And the news gets even better.

Snack in the Middle

NOT ONLY CAN YOU enjoy your three main meals — plus dessert — but you can also treat yourself to a host of nourishing nibbles throughout the day. While this certainly doesn't mean that you should binge — there can be too much of a good thing — snacking has its merits. Here's a look at some interesting facts:

- Eating several mini-meals a day keeps energy levels from slumping.

- If you're trying to lose weight, "grazing" on healthy foods throughout the day keeps you feeling satisfied, and keeps your metabolism revved up.

- Healthy nibbling reduces the demand on your digestive system, burning off calories as you go on working. The trick is to keep portions quite small.

- Snacking spices things up. The long-lived Japanese recommend eating up to thirty different foods as part of a few mini-meals per day to prevent overeating any one item and to get a variety of nutrients in your diet.

That is why I snack throughout the day — on oranges, grapes, light pretzels, hot-air popcorn, organic yogurt, carrots, raisins, and, occasionally, a small bar of chocolate. Inspired by my friend Sylvia's plentiful pantry, I've created my own treasure trove of nourishing nibbles. Can't wait to do the same? Delve into the delicious world of snack ideas that await you on the website www.healthycookingrecipes.com.

Tuck healthful bites in easy-to-reach places, such as:

- Your purse: dark chocolate or fruit. (Dark chocolate contains beneficial antioxidants, so go ahead and eat a bar once in a while.)
- Your briefcase: sachets of herb tea, packets of popcorn.
- Your glove compartment: nuts, trail mix, dried fruit.
- Your office refrigerator: soy milk, baby carrots, cottage cheese, hummus.
- Your desk drawer: whole-grain crackers, baked corn chips.

Don't forget to keep these areas clean and critter-proof!

The Pleasure of It All

NOW THAT WE'VE DISCUSSED weighty matters such as the quality, quantity, and health benefits of what we eat, there remains one aspect to consider, without which any talk of food is incomplete. That aspect is enjoyment! Yes, food is fuel and energy, but above all, it is — and happily so — a prime source of pleasure and contentment. So, in the daily grind of life, don't forget to slow down once in a while and allow yourself to luxuriate in the many flavors of your life. As I say this, I'm thinking of that wonderful time we get at the end of every five days: the weekend. This regular interlude can be the perfect opportunity for you to discover the many pleasures of connecting with food and family.

Here are some succulent suggestions for an unhurried day:

Curl Up with a Cookbook

THERE'S SOMETHING MAGICAL about seeing these instructions in print:

- Fold in the fruit.

- Bake until crisp-tender.

- Serve warm, with clotted cream or honey.

Have you ever curled up in your favorite bay window with a beautifully illustrated cookbook instead of a novel? I do it all the time. A good cookbook gives you more than recipes; it invites you into the ambrosial world of flavor, it whets your appetite, and it lets your imagination run wild.

Just last evening, I was reading a book about Mediterranean cooking. As I savored the recipes for *tapas* and *mezze*, my eyes lingered pleasurably on the photographs with their brilliant blue plates, bright green-and-orange salads, red-and-white napkins, and shapely oil bottles. Soon I was so involved that I could almost smell the aroma of the ingredients rising off the pages — crusty bread, sun-ripened tomatoes, toasted pine nuts — thrilling my

---

GHEE

Ghee, or clarified butter, is a delicious and healthy alternative to store-bought butter. You will find ghee in most Indian food recipes, and you can make it quite easily at home. Here's how:

> Take 1 pound cultured, unsalted organic butter and place it in a medium saucepan and slowly melt over medium heat. When the butter comes to a boil, reduce the heat and simmer the butter uncovered and undisturbed for 45 to 60 minutes. As the temperature reaches the boiling point of water, the butter's water content vaporizes and the butter foams and makes tiny, sharp, crackling noises. The milk solids in the butter will slowly settle to the bottom, leaving pale golden liquid on top that you can sieve immediately into a clean glass jar. This is ghee. Ghee stays fresh for a few weeks at room temperature. You might, however, want to refrigerate it.

taste buds and propelling me toward the kitchen. Instead of the soup and bread I had planned, I ended up cooking grilled vegetables with ricotta cheese and lemon dressing — much to the pleasant surprise of my family.

Dine in Style

WE HAVE A SAYING IN INDIA: *Ghar ki murgi dal barabar.* That is, "If it is cooked at home, even a luscious chicken dish can seem as unappetizing as simple lentils." That's because, at home, we hardly ever take the trouble to dress up our dining table or create an appetizing ambience.

Restaurant designers, on the other hand, know exactly how to cater to our five senses. The appetite-enhancing reds and yellows on the wall, those flowers and candles on your table, the dim lighting, the sliver of lime afloat in your glass of water, the menu cards with their poetic descriptions of food ("Oven-simmered lentils cooked with spices and smothered in fresh cream..."). Together, they serenade your senses until your taste buds tingle and your body readies itself to enjoy the meal — even if it is a sandwich you could have put together at home for one-fourth the price. Steal their ideas! Such creative touches as flowers, candles, and garnishes are inexpensive but lots of fun to do. As for the menu card, I've tried

> ### ONE MANTRA TO REMEMBER WHEN YOU COOK
>
> Keep it simple. Let the word "simple" be an acronym for:
>
> **S**mall portions
>
> **I**ntuitive eating
>
> **M**indful shopping
>
> **P**leasant ambience
>
> **L**oving preparation and
>
> **E**legant presentation
>
> That's all you need to make a meal truly healing and wholesome.

it and it perks up the atmosphere beautifully. I have a simple blackboard in my kitchen, announcing "Today's Special" in colored chalk. Even if it is a simple dish of baked potatoes, I call it "freshly baked potatoes bursting with butter and flavor." It's a cheerful touch, and it inspires me to make whatever I do with more love.

Play with Your Food

THESE DAYS, I'm reading an interesting book by Tom Colicchio. It's called *Think Like a Chef.* In the introduction, Chef Colicchio says, "I don't sit down and 'create' food combinations. I start in the marketplace, walking…What's abundant? What's growing together naturally? Which herbs are peaking? Above all, what are the seasons saying? What I see starts me thinking about flavors and textures, combinations and balance."[2] I am sure the secret of this man's success as a chef is in his natural, playful approach to food. He creates from the heart, exploring new flavors, new combinations, and new worlds.

On Saturdays, cook ordinary ingredients in fresh ways. For instance, if you've always eaten your spuds mashed or baked or fried, let me invite you to discover potatoes cooked the Indian way. They are simply delicious eaten with warm bread.

SPICY POTATOES

2 tablespoons olive oil or ghee

1/2 teaspoon cumin seeds

1 purple onion, finely sliced

3 cloves garlic, minced

1/2-inch piece of fresh ginger root, minced

1 medium-sized tomato, finely sliced

1 cup plain nonfat yogurt, whisked until smooth

1/2 teaspoon turmeric powder

salt to taste

3 russet potatoes, washed and cubed

2 cups water

1/2 teaspoon garam masala (hot spice mix available at
    Indian grocery stores)

a bunch of freshly chopped cilantro leaves

Heat oil or ghee (see sidebar on page 54 for recipe) in a medium-sized pan. When the oil is medium-hot, put in the cumin seeds. As soon as the seeds begin to crackle (this will take just a few seconds), add the onion, garlic, and ginger. Sauté for a few minutes until the mixture turns a golden brown. Now put in the tomatoes, yogurt, turmeric, and salt. Cook until the oil separates from the paste (you'll see it bubbling on the sides). Add the cubed potatoes and stir to coat them well with the paste. Pour in the water and cover the vessel. Simmer the potatoes for about 20 minutes, or until completely cooked. Add garam masala and cilantro, and serve hot. Makes 4 servings.

For an interesting variation, you can add a cup of chopped cauliflower, green peas, or finely sliced cabbage to this recipe.

Similarly, find new ways to cook with herbs. Think

HOW TO IGNITE YOUR APPETITE

- Have open shelving in your kitchen. Show off those jars, brimming with cereals and grains.

- Bring all those fruits and fresh vegetables out of the fridge and mound them in colorful — or just plain white — bowls.

- Arrange fresh herbs — chives, parsley, and cilantro — like bouquets in tall glasses half-filled with fresh, cool water.

beyond chives and sage. Wake up your sleepy salads with herbs like red basil, purple orach, bronze fennel, or chicory leaves. Dill weed adds an exciting twist to salad, and rosemary, traditionally recommended for use with potatoes, is equally egg-citing on scrambled eggs. Also, did you know that some flowers could be absolutely delicious? Marigold has a piquant taste and smell. Bergamot has a rich oriental fragrance. Nasturtiums are sweet, spicy, and colorful. Chamomile flowers are lovely in tea. Chive blossoms bring an oniony taste and smell.

> **FIVE DELICIOUS DINNERTIME MOVIES**
> ....
> *Chocolat*
>
> *Fried Green Tomatoes*
>
> *Like Water for Chocolate*
>
> *Mystic Pizza*
>
> *Tortilla Soup*

This week, it's herbs. Next week, work — no, play — with spices. Then the Saturday after that, explore the succulent world of fruits, or grains, or sauces.

Once a Month, Create a Memorable Meal

IF YOU STICK TO a well-balanced, healthy diet most of the time, allow yourself to indulge in a rich treat once in a while. Pick out one night every four weeks to enjoy an old family favorite, without worrying about the calories. Let that meal become more than a sensory indulgence — make it an occasion for you to bond with those you love. I read this quotation somewhere many years ago: "Even baking a cake is a spiritual thing, for you are serving someone." It's easy to buy cake from your local supermarket, but the truth is that your children will never forget homemade cakes, made from scratch and made with love. So make friends with your oven. Start by baking the simplest angel cake or pound cake, then go on to more interesting ones, such as Upside-Down Apple Cake,

Tyrolean Coffee Gateau, and Black Forest Trifle. Ask your friends for recipes, join a cooking school, or try recipes from a book. What a joy it is to watch the warm cake disappear within minutes of emerging from the oven!

Thinking back to my own bountiful days of childhood, the images are still so fresh that I can almost smell the lemons as my aunt slices them on the verandah for pickling with turmeric and fenugreek. Or my mother, freshly bathed, salutes the threshold before entering the kitchen first thing in the morning. Soon her gentle voice will say, "Come children, settle down on the *chatai* (straw mat); I've cooked your favorite curried potatoes and okra today." And the most vivid image of them all: my grandmother vigorously churning fresh buttermilk in a pot, while singing this endearingly mean poem (I'm translating from Hindi):

> *The rich young woman's son is bawling,*
> *Clinging to her sari silk,*
> *Let him bawl, let him yell,*
> *But let me churn my buttermilk,*
> *jhakkar jhoon ah! jhakkar jhoon.*
> *Jhakkar jhoon ah! jhakkar jhoon.*

"Jhakkar jhoon" is almost exactly the sound that grandma's wooden whisk made as it rotated deep in the belly of the earthen pot. Of course, the sentiment behind the words was never to ignore a bawling child — grandma was too tender for that — but to cherish the moment of stirring the buttermilk.

With grandma's song still echoing in my heart, I'll leave you to savor the nourishing thoughts I've shared with you. I hope they leave a good, lingering aftertaste in your heart. Meanwhile, I'll go treat myself to a warm bath. I have a delicious evening to look forward to: We're invited to dinner at my friend Sylvia's!

THOUGHTS FROM HANNAH POLMER,
JEWELRY DESIGNER, 40

My kitchen is a sacred place: the heart of our home. Most of my creative endeavors happen in this space. I've got a palette of ingredients to choose from and two hands to create the most eye-pleasing, aromatic sensations.

After a stressful day, working with my hands chopping vegetables, kneading pastry dough, squishing lemons, or smelling aromatic spices exploding into the heat of water or oil brings me back to life and into a moment of creating infinite possibilities. I can stare into a pot of risotto while stirring, thinking of nothing else but the beauty of its creamy texture. The repetitive motion can also calm my thoughts to help resolve pressing issues accumulated throughout the day. I believe it's art — this beautiful creation. There is so much joy and comfort in the whole experience, from beginning to end.

Throughout the winter months, I love to prepare stews and soups because of the mixture of flavors I can create on the stovetop. The aroma permeates my house and brings warmth and comfort to us, as well as to anyone visiting for dinner.

The following vegetable soup with pesto is a great winter dish. One may also choose to use it as a base (without pesto) for a curry soup with lentils or other beans.

Vegetable Soup with Pesto

1½ cup onions

1½ cup celery

2 cups scallions or leeks

1 green pepper

Several tablespoons olive oil

9 cups water

1 tablespoon salt

1¹/₂ cups carrots

1¹/₂ cups butternut squash

1¹/₂ cups potatoes

1¹/₂ cups zucchini

1 cup string beans

1 cup lettuce leaves

2 cups spinach

Pesto

1 cup basil leaves

4 cloves garlic

¹/₄ cup Parmesan cheese

¹/₄ cup olive oil

Chop vegetables into ¹/₂ inch pieces, except for the lettuce and spinach. They can be left whole or cut in half, if desired.

Sauté onions, celery, scallions, and green pepper in olive oil for several minutes. Add water, salt, and remaining vegetables, except for the lettuce and spinach. Bring to a boil. Lower the heat, cover, and simmer for approximately 30 minutes. Add lettuce and spinach and simmer for approximately 15 minutes.

Meanwhile, prepare the pesto by puréeing all the ingredients in a food processor or blender until smooth. When the soup is cooked, stir in the pesto and serve.

I prefer baked fruit desserts during winter months. A fruit cobbler is a perfect excuse to dive right in, use your hands, feel the texture of the flour and butter together, and make something scrumptious.

During the summer months, a cold fruit salad is a tempting treat with fresh mint, ginger, and rosewater added to cool and soothe the senses after an active day in the sun. I usually have cold fruit drinks stored in the refrigerator, such as this one:

Watermelon Cooler

Mix several tablespoons of sugar with spring water in a pitcher. Add approximately 2 cups of watermelon cut into small cubes, a handful of fresh mint, and the juice of one or more limes; refrigerate. Pour into individual glasses when cool, and garnish with melon slices. Delicious!

Chapter Summary and Resources

- Every woman represents Annapoorna, the Hindu goddess of nourishment. You can be an Annapoorna, too, no matter how hectic your life.

- Good nutrition begins with intelligent grocery shopping. Almost every issue of magazines such as *Family Circle, First for Women,* and *Woman's Day* carries tips for clever grocery shopping; jot down those you find useful. In addition, ask your friends to share their healthy-shopping secrets. Three golden tips I've learned:

  1. Never shop for food on an empty stomach.

  2. Always shop with a grocery list.

  3. Avoid taking kids to the supermarket so that you're not persuaded to buy fat-laden cookies and chips.

- Get a head start on your day: Eat a good breakfast. For a feast of ideas on how to make your mornings special, read *The Good Enough to Eat Breakfast Cookbook* by Carrie Levin (Warner Books, 2001). It's a sumptuous selection, best enjoyed on your couch in the evening so that you can plan your menu for the next morning.

- Appetite and energy — both peak at noon. So make lunch your main meal of the day.

- Keep dinner light. You'll sleep more easily, and you'll wake up with a healthy appetite for breakfast.

- Can you have your cake and eat it, too? Yes! Delve into the world of delicious desserts that don't go straight to your hips.

- Nibble, nibble. Light snacking at regular intervals keeps your metabolism active and stops you from overeating.

- A good cookbook is a window to the varied world of culture and cuisine. Take time to savor a cookbook on a relaxed afternoon. There's a dazzling array of books about nutrition out there, but my personal favorite is Miriam Kasin Hospodar's *Heaven's Banquet.* This sumptuous book will introduce you to traditional Indian cuisine — pure, natural, and intuitive — in a light, entertaining manner. You'll find hundreds of succulent vegetarian recipes, as well as food quotations and humor sprinkled throughout its 390 pages.

- Give your home a restaurant-like ambience with simple touches such as a menu handwritten on blackboard, a table set with style, and food served on your best china. Look for ideas on television shows, such as *Decorating on a Dime,* and bring back ideas from your favorite restaurant next time you dine there.

- The world of food can be greatly creative! Always try new flavors and look for ways to perk up old recipes. Serious about good cooking? Take a short course! The renowned French Culinary Institute in New York City offers a forty-hour course for amateur cooks. Called "Essentials of Fine Cooking," the course is "for everyone from noncooks to sophisticated home cooks who want to raise the level of their culinary skills and cook delicious, beautiful food at home." For more information, log on to www.frenchculinary.com. Every summer, *Food and Wine* magazine holds an exciting food festival in the mountain resort of Aspen, Colorado, where America's top chefs gather and attendees get to sample delicious food and learn luscious cooking secrets. Surf the Internet for dozens of other exciting food workshops and festivals.

CHAPTER 3

Beauty

How to Be Lovelier — Inside and Out

Won't you come into the garden? I would like my roses to see you.
— RICHARD BRINSLEY SHERIDAN

*N*amaste. The word means: "I salute the divine in you." This is how the people of India greet each other, with palms joined together in a gesture of respect. The greeting stems from the deep Hindu belief that inside each of us is a place where truth, beauty, light, and love reside.

Don't you think that such a beautiful belief deserves to transcend the barriers of religion and weave itself into our lives and culture? Not the words or the greeting — just the belief. What a difference it will make in the way we look at others and, indeed, at ourselves.

The Error of the Mirror

THEY SAY MIRRORS DON'T LIE. They are right — but only to an extent. A mirror can be mistaken. If a mirror is telling us that we look less than lovely, it is mistaken because it is making us feel apologetic for not being slender, svelte, and sexy like those movie stars and models we see all the time. Result: We forget our connection with the Divine, and we begin to believe that we are, indeed, unbeautiful. Ancient sages of India had a Sanskrit term for this: *pragya aparadh* — mistake of the intellect.

Correct this mistake! Think of yourself as a magnificent part of nature, just like the lovely dewdrop, the sunset, and the rose. Ask yourself how boring the world would be if every woman had Cindy Crawford's face and mole and figure. What makes life beautiful is its variety and spice — and your unique looks are a joyous part of that smorgasbord.

Even so, the urge to look and feel her best is natural to woman, and why not? Working toward looking physically attractive isn't always a sign of vanity. It shows that you love and respect the body you inhabit, and that is a very gracious thing to do.

Congratulations! You have the power to look gorgeous without going under the plastic surgeon's knife or checking into an expensive spa. What's more, it's never too late — or too early — to begin your quest for renewal. All you have to do is allow yourself time to enjoy some simple self-care rituals.

You Are *a Star*

READY TO WIPE THAT DUST off the surface of your intellect? Wonderful! In small, simple steps, let's walk back to the true, beautiful, radiant, lovely place inside of you. Start with these building blocks of a positive self-image:

Befriend Your Body

A SWEET-SMELLING BODY, fresh breath, and clean clothes — they're guaranteed to make you feel self-confident and comfortable. Therefore:

Maintain good hygiene at all times. Bathe daily. Bathing is not only a pleasurable personal ritual, it is essential for shedding pollutants, chemicals, and lethargy from your body and mind. Even if your schedule allows you nothing but a hurried shower, make it a point to clean your body every day. While bathing, pay special attention to the temperature of the water — if it causes condensation on the bathroom mirror, it is too warm, and if it gives you goosebumps, it is too cold. Healers in India advise waiting a few minutes after a meal, sexual activity, exercise, or massage to allow the body to come back to its normal temperature before you go in for a shower or bath. As you rinse away the dirt and dust, paying special attention to areas such as feet and underarms, don't forget to sing in the shower — it's a great way to release tension!

After your bath, take care to dry the groin; women are prone to vaginal infections, so use your hair dryer on a cool setting to dry this area thoroughly after a bath. Also, towel-dry your armpits, between your toes, and behind your knees thoroughly to prevent odor-causing bacteria from building up.

Keep your mouth smelling clean and fresh at all times. Brush and floss twice daily; this might sound like trivial advice, but it is basic to your good health and confidence. Rinse your mouth thoroughly after every meal and, preferably, after every cup of tea or coffee, too. Chew on carrots and apples to give your jaws a workout, freshen your breath, and get some nourishment in the bargain. My grandmother, who retained her strong original teeth into her nineties, would massage her gums daily with a circulation-boosting paste of mustard oil and finely ground rock salt. Try it, and I promise your gums will feel tighter and look healthier within a week of regular use. To make the paste, pour out a teaspoon of mustard oil — you can also use clove oil — into a cupped palm. Take a generous pinch of the salt and mix it into the oil with the index finger of your other hand. Then, using your index finger, gently rub this paste in an up-and-down motion on your gums every morning after brushing. Rinse out with water. Here's another way to disinfect your mouth and freshen your breath: Chew mint leaves. Chewing sugarless gum is a good way to encourage saliva flow and keep your breath smelling clean. Visit your dentist regularly. If you have an uneven bite or stained teeth, ask how they can be corrected; dental procedures today are not only advanced, they are virtually painless.

Rethink the way you shop for clothes. Do you tend to buy on impulse, to lift your mood, or just because there is a sale? If so, chances are that you're saddled with a lot of outfits that you don't wear often or that don't make you feel especially good. Here's an easy fix: Give away the items that are languishing in your closet and make room for clothes that you would love to wear again and again. Make this de-cluttering exercise fun; get together with a friend and model your clothes for her. Ask her to be brutally honest and help you decide which ones to keep and which to discard. Do the same for your friend. Once you have a clear picture of the items you need to complete your wardrobe, go ahead and do some sensible, enjoyable clothes shopping. You don't need to buy twenty new dresses to look good; the key is to own a few classic pieces, accessorize them well, and care for them.

Take another look at your shoes. Do they reflect a preference for high heels? If yes, here is some down-to-earth advice: High heels may look stylish, but they force the front portion of your feet to bear the entire weight of your body, distorting your posture. If you must wear high heels, reserve them for special occasions. For regular use, buy comfortable, flat-heeled shoes — there's a dazzling variety of them out there — and walk naturally tall. A few tips for choosing the right shoe: Make sure it matches the shape of your foot, doesn't feel too snug or too loose, and supports the ball of your foot in a comfortable hug. Shoe shopping should never be a hurried, uncertain affair. Don't let a salesperson coax you into buying a pair on the promise that it will stretch with use. Walk around in the store to judge whether your feet like the feel of the shoes.

Walk straight. Have you ever met a lovely person who slouches or slumps? An upright posture is graceful, helps avoid muscle aches and pains, and spells self-confidence. Project a calm personality: Don't fiddle with your buttons, clothes, or hair. Don't bite your nails, doodle aimlessly, or drum your fingers on the table; these gestures rob you of grace and charm.

FIVE BEAUTIFUL GIFTS
YOU CAN GIVE TO YOUR BODY

1. **The gift of acceptance:** Stop climbing on and off those scales! Don't fret constantly over that strand of gray hair, those crow's feet, and the half-inch increase in your waist. And so what if your colleague has a figure to die for? Live life queen-size in the body you have.

2. **The gift of listening:** When you're hungry, eat. When you're full, stop. When your eyes ache with strain, shut down the computer. Honor your body's needs, and it will glow.

3. **The gift of pride:** Carry yourself with grace. Walk tall. Hold your head high. Sit erect.

4. **The gift of good maintenance:** Get an annual eye exam and a dental check-up every six months. Once in a while, treat yourself to a good detoxifying and cleansing diet; this gives your entire system much-needed rest and replenishment.

5. **The gift of comfort:** Don't squeeze your frame into a dress that is tight at the waist. Never force your feet into ill-fitting shoes. Wear clothes that are comfortable, fit you well, and suit the season. If you work long hours at the computer, take care to use an ergonomically designed chair, and provide adequate support to your wrists and your back.

Make Over Your Mind

THE MIND INTERPRETS and responds to signals that your five senses send it. If those signals are negative, your mind-set grows negative, too. The solution is to filter out the negative signals from your life. Start looking for them, and you'll find that there are many!

- If you refuse to wear a swimsuit because you don't have the figure of a *Baywatch* babe, it's time to stop watching TV shows and advertisements that generate feelings of inferiority. Choose your reading material carefully, too. If *Cosmo* gals make you rue your figure, subscribe to *Self*. I also like *Glamour* magazine which, despite its name, always includes an article about how to love your body just the way it is.

- Are you anorexic, bulimic, or a yo-yo dieter? If so, don't delay! Read up on the harmful effects of these drastic "beauty" measures. You'll soon realize that they will not only diminish your looks, but also wreck your digestive system and make you sick.

- Do you have friends who obsess about their looks and comment on yours all the time? If so, spend a few evenings with them reassessing your attitudes as a group. Share success stories of women who are known as beautiful for their energy, radiance, and goodness of heart. Think about ways to be beautiful from the inside out by improving your diet and lifestyle. If your friends refuse to support your desire to look at things in a more positive way, you might want to reassess the company you keep.

- Do something you're especially good at. If you're a good cook, make a wonderful dish and invite someone home to share it with you. If you paint, create a work of art and display it in a special corner of your home. If it's writing that lights your fire, play wordsmith. Doing something well fills you with a sense of achievement that goes beyond the physical. You don't have to prove anything to anyone; as long as it makes you feel happy and fulfilled, a creative activity is its own reward.

• "Don't postpone joy," says H. Jackson Brown in the ever-popular *Life's Little Instruction Book.*[1] Follow its advice. Romance the rain. Take a walk in the snow; feel it going "crunch-crunch" under your feet. Sip coffee on the deck with your best friend. Do anything that brings your heart joy, and you'll glow.

• Be nice! Smile! It's the easiest makeover you can give yourself. Be generous with compliments. Do a good deed every day. The beauty of a kind face is natural and pure.

Of course, there are times when one cannot help feeling low. It could be as trivial as a bad hair day, or as disturbing as the breakup of a relationship. You might be feeling overweight, or there may be frustrations at work or at home. When you find yourself swamped by such feelings, take some quiet time to contemplate the following beautiful, healing words of wise sages.

> *Beauty is an ecstasy; it is as simple as hunger. There is really nothing to be said about it. It is like the perfume of a rose: you can smell it and that is all.*
> — W. Somerset Maugham

> *We ask ourselves, who are we to be brilliant, gorgeous, talented and fabulous? Actually, who are we not to be?*
> — Marianne Williamson

> *Beauty of style and harmony and grace and good rhythm*
> *depend on simplicity.*
>
> — Plato

> *Exuberance is beauty.*
>
> — William Blake

Write these words in your personal diary, or frame them. Find your own special quotes, or write down your own thoughts and feelings about what makes you feel beautiful.

❈

OF COURSE, you cannot make all these mind-body changes in one go. Begin with the one you find easiest, or one that you feel really needs attention. It could be observing better oral hygiene or

---

FEEL BEAUTIFUL NOW!

"NOW" is a beautiful word:

N is for Nutrition

O is for Oxygen

W is for Water

Just once a day, give yourself the NOW check; it's an easy, instant way to connect with your body.

Let's do it right NOW. Close this book and ask your body which of these it wants: food, air, or water. The body, which loves to communicate with you, will respond at once. Go ahead: Treat yourself to some good food or a light snack, take a few deep breaths or a brief stroll for fresh air, or enjoy a tall glass of water or squeeze yourself some juice.

This simple act of kindness will keep you feeling loved — and lovely — throughout the day.

making positive affirmations. Whatever you choose to do, don't load yourself with expectations. In time, the layer of dust on your intellect is sure to dissipate, allowing you to feel naturally radiant.

Now I'll introduce you to my favorite body-beautiful tips. Not only will they make you glow on the outside, but they'll also suffuse you with inner radiance.

The Healing Touch

I'M TALKING ABOUT MASSAGE. If you haven't yet discovered the magic of self-massage, welcome to the world of refreshing rub-downs. It never ceases to amaze me how something as simple as rubbing oil over your skin can do so much for your mind, body, and spirit. Here's a list of the most basic benefits of massage:

- It isn't the oils and creams used in massage that make it so special; it's the sense of touch. A woman needs to be touched with love, and when you smooth warm oil all over your body, you satisfy that basic feminine need. Giving or receiving a massage is one of the luxuries of life; done with tenderness and good technique, it is often a delicious prelude to making love.

- Up and down, slow and smooth, warm and wicked — the rhythms of massage have a way of seducing the stress out of your system. As for your skin, what could it love more than the moisture and sheen it receives from well-oiled hands?

- Infused with healing herbs, such as brahmi, ashwa-gandha, rosemary, or lavender, massage oil nourishes body tissue from deep within.

- Massage improves circulation, sending a fresh supply of oxygen to your cells. This relaxes muscles that have been tense from a day of hard work, soothes and lubricates the joints, and speeds up the removal of toxic debris from your system.

• In the long run, regular massage maintains the youthfulness of skin, keeping it lustrous and healthy throughout your life.

Massage Made Easy

ARE YOU TEMPTED TO TRY out self-massage now? Here's how to do it:

What You Need for a Knead

BUY "CURED" OR PURIFIED OIL from a natural food store. Choose among sesame, almond, and olive oil; they suit all types of skin. Choose cold-pressed, chemical-free, organic brands for a pure-bliss experience.

For an even more healing experience, you can infuse your massage oil with herbs. It's easy to do. Using your palms or a rolling pin, crush a handful of dried herbs — rosemary, lemon verbena, bergamot, calendula, chamomile, or lavender — to help them release their oils. Stir them into your massage oil, then let the oil stand for a few days. Make small quantities at a time — say, one and a half cups — enough to last two to three days. Refrigerate the portion you are not using right away. When your first bottle of infused oil is ready, start another batch. Alternatively, buy a good-quality herb-infused oil from a natural products store.

When you're ready to begin your massage, set the bottle of oil into a pan or container of hot water. Allow the bottle to stand in the hot water until it is warmed throughout to body temperature or just a little warmer. Make sure the oil is not too hot or uncomfortable to the touch. Warming the oil helps it penetrate skin better and feels more comforting.

Rubbing It In

TAKE OFF YOUR CLOTHES and sit comfortably on an old towel by your bathtub. Pour a small quantity of the warm oil into your palm and dip the fingertips of your free hand into the oil. Lightly apply the oil all over your scalp, face, torso, arms, legs, and feet. Once you've covered every inch of your skin with a light layer of oil, pour some more oil into a bowl. Dip your fingertips in the bowl, and begin massaging each area of your body in flat-handed strokes, starting with the scalp.

Different Strokes

SCALP: USING YOUR FINGERTIPS, massage your scalp in a circular motion, moving in an arc from the top of your head downward to the base of your neck.

REFRESHING FIVE-MINUTE SELF-MASSAGE

Use a good-quality organic lotion for this massage. Squeeze some lotion onto the palm of one hand. Dip the pads of the fingers of your other hand in the lotion, and gently tap your face with them. The lotion will be dotted across your face, and the tapping action will wake up tired skin. Now use slow, circular motions to spread the lotion on your face with the same fingers.

Using the same technique, massage your arms, legs, and feet with the lotion. Use circular strokes on the joints — such as ankles, knees, and elbows — and long, firm strokes along your limbs.

This quick, simple massage will quench your skin's thirst for moisture, and leave you feeling young and fragrant within minutes.

Limbs: Rub your fingers lengthwise along your arms and legs, and in a gentle circular motion on joints such as elbows, knees, and ankles.

Points of bliss: Pay special attention to areas where nerve endings are concentrated, such as the soles of your feet, your earlobes, the hollows of your temples, and the center of the underside of your wrist.

Take care: Soften the pressure when you're oiling sensitive areas, such as your abdomen, breasts, and heart area.

After Your Massage

WHEN YOU'RE THROUGH with your massage, relax for about twenty minutes, if time permits. This allows the oil to penetrate deep into your tissues, and your mind to feel settled. You can read a good book, listen to soothing music, or simply lie on the floor in your bedroom (keeping the towel underneath your body, of course).

When you're through relaxing, wipe off any excess oil from your skin with the towel, and enjoy a warm shower or bath. It is essential to wash the oil off your body so that it doesn't clog your pores. Use a mild, oil-based herbal soap. Don't use harsh soap after your massage, because the detergent will leach the oil from your pores. If your skin is not very sensitive, you can also use barley or chickpea flour to gently lift the oil — and with it, dead cells — from the surface of your skin. Always hand-wash the oily towel afterward to avoid the risk of the washing machine catching fire.

Done this way, self-massage will take approximately an hour from start to finish, including time in the shower. This is perfect for an unhurried Saturday morning when you're in the mood to do something restorative for yourself. This mmm-massage hour will coax the tiredness out of your skin and your very spirits, renewing you for the week ahead.

But hey, don't feel that you can't massage yourself every day! If your day is impossibly hectic, try squeezing in three to five minutes for a quick massage before your shower. Just make your strokes quicker, and shorten the gap between massage and shower.

The Magic of a Five-Minute Massage

LOOK AT THE BENEFITS this small investment of your time will yield: Within five days of massaging your body — even for five minutes a day — you'll notice happy changes in the way you look and feel. Your skin will feel supple and smooth, thanks to the oil that has nourished its deeper layers in these five days. Lubricated by warm, herb-infused oil, your joints and muscles will feel more flexible and relaxed. The actions of gently rubbing, stroking, and kneading — even if done for a short while — give your circulation a boost. You'll therefore find yourself feeling more alert and motivated throughout the day. With all these good things happening to your body, your heart will hum, too.

The After-Massage Soak

LIKE YOUR BEDROOM, your bathing space is a personal sanctuary. Here, insulated from the world, you are free to spend time with the body you live inside. Stretch it, scrub it, relax it, cleanse it, and pamper it. In the process, do something you've longed to do all day: Connect with yourself.

Sylvia Plath once wrote, "There must be quite a few things a hot bath won't cure, but I don't know many of them."[2] Plunge into a warm tub tonight, and you'll agree.

A Warming Ginger Bath

HERE'S A DELICIOUS post-massage soak to try:

What it will do for you: soothe aching joints; warm your body; coax your day's stress away; make you look, smell, and feel like a queen.

Before your bath: Make a comfortable bed, with clean sheets and cozy pillows. Dim the lights and set out aromatherapy candles by your bedside. Since you should never leave a burning candle unattended, light the candles after you return from your bath and enjoy their soothing essence as it permeates the air. You could also spritz your sheets with a mix of water and essential oil, or put some rosewater in a bowl next to your bed so that a lovely, soothing fragrance will greet you when you snuggle in.

Bath essentials: fresh ginger root; a bath oil of your choice; body lotion of your choice; body mist (store-bought or made at home by stirring a few drops of your favorite essential oil into a bottle of clean water); a large, clean towel; your favorite music; a glass of chilled wine or water with a few slices of fresh cucumber floating in it; a fluffy bathrobe; snug bath slippers; and comfortable night clothes.

The bath: Begin to play your favorite music. Slice a small piece of ginger lengthwise, leaving the skin on. Drop it in boiling water and let it simmer for about fifteen minutes. Tuck your hair into a shower cap. Run your bath water. While the tub fills up, cleanse your face and neck using a homemade fruit pack (see recipes, page 82) or a natural, organic one purchased from a health store. Set your glass of wine or cucumber water beside the tub. Pour the ginger, along with the water it was boiled in, into the bathtub. Test the water temperature for comfort. Step in, lie back, and stretch your limbs until a delectable languor settles in. With the music on and your drink trailing seductively down your throat, the world and its problems will slowly recede from your mind. At this time, you can gently run a loofah over your body to stimulate your skin and rid it of dead cells. Afterward, pat your skin dry with your towel, mist rosewater or lavender water all over your body, and gently massage body lotion into your arms, legs, feet, shoulders — everywhere you can reach.

Head off to bed, and feel the slumber kiss your eyes.

Introducing the World's Best Cosmetics Factory

IN 1739, a man named Pierre Joseph Buc'hoz wrote a book called *The Toilet of Flora*. The book was described as "A Collection of the Most Simple and Approved Methods of Preparing Baths, Essences, Pomatums, Powders, Perfumes, and Sweet-Scented Waters. With Recipes for Cosmetics of every kind, that can smooth and brighten the Skin, give Force to Beauty, and take off the Appearance of Old Age and Decay. For The Use Of The Ladies."

Today the book is worth nearly $2,000, but the advice in it is worth millions. In it, Buc'hoz discussed ways to make beauty masks and lotions from simple kitchen ingredients. Take a page from Buc'hoz's precious beauty book. We've come a long way since then, but our kitchen still remains a treasure-house of ingredients that can give your skin everything it needs: moisture, conditioning, toning, exfoliation, cleansing, rejuvenation, and radiance. Once you start to play cosmetic-maker, you won't want to stop!

Five Reasons to Make Cosmetics at Home

- You are what you eat, and your skin is what it absorbs. The seven million pores on your skin, which release oil and sweat, also take in what you put on the surface. This means that rubbing a cream on your arms is as good (or as bad) as eating the chemicals in it.

- Even so-called organic, natural beauty products can contain undesirable, unrevealed chemicals.

- Homemade cosmetics are less expensive and more fun than store-bought ones.

- Creating your own packs and masks puts you more intimately in touch with what your skin needs and likes.

- Being your own beautician gives you a sense of self-esteem and joy that comes from spending time on yourself.

And now, let me share with you some super, simple ideas for homemade skin-pampering packs.

The Skin-Sational Kitchen

THIS WEEKEND, delve into your pantry and your fridge for ingredients you can use on your skin. You'll find scores of them. It's perfectly okay to experiment with fruits, vegetables, nuts, seeds, and oils, as long as you observe this rule of thumb: If it is safe enough to eat, it is safe enough to apply on skin. Take care: Avoid ingredients that you are allergic to; if you're not sure, make a tiny amount of a pack and try it on a small patch of skin to see if a reaction occurs.

Here are some ideas about how you can give yourself salon-quality care in five minutes a day:

Frequent-Use Fruit Pack

SIMPLE FRUIT PULP is rich in vitamin A and beta-carotene, and a nourishing fruit pack is easy to make. Peel and mash a ripe organic mango (nonorganic fruit usually contains pesticides and chemicals, which can seep into your skin through your pores). If you don't have mangoes at home, you can try a papaya, an avocado, three strawberries, half a banana — whatever you've got in your fridge or your fruit bowl. Apply two teaspoons of the pulp to your face. Five to seven minutes later, wash your face with warm water and pat it dry. Enjoy the rest of the fruit for dessert! Now this is what I call nourishing the skin from the inside out. This soft, luscious pack can be safely used every day.

Another variation is to finely grate a carrot or banana, add one to two teaspoons of milk, and apply it to your face. Yum!

Eye-Fatigue Fighter

SEND UNDER-EYE BAGS packing with the help of — you'll never guess — a spud! Potatoes are rich in vitamin K, which has a known role in dispersing collected fluids that cause puffiness. It also lightens dark patches on the skin. Next time you make hash browns, set aside a tablespoon of grated raw potatoes. While the golden treat cooks, lie back with the grated spuds applied to those under-eye bags. Remove the potatoes gently after a few minutes, and wipe the area delicately with a warm towel. If your skin is particularly sensitive, wash the potato juice off your skin with warm water. Use this potato-soother after a long day, when your eyes feel tired.

Rich-But-Inexpensive Night Cream

SOME OF THE NIGHT CREAMS you can buy are very effective, no doubt, but they're also expensive. Here's how to make your own from a handful of almonds. Next time you boil pasta, don't drain the water away; use it to blanch a handful of shelled organic almonds. The hot water will enable the brown skins to slide off the almonds easily. Leave the blanched almonds in the refrigerator overnight, then grind them with about three

A FLOUR FIT FOR QUEENS

You may have heard exotic tales of how queens in ancient India bathed — using gold dust, sandalwood, turmeric, milk, and rose petals. Fast-forward a few centuries. Women in India still love natural ingredients, but they have discovered several less expensive and equally effective alternatives to gold and fragrant woods.

One such ingredient is "gram flour," which is made from dried chickpeas. Used for making curries and fritters, it is absolutely delicious and protein-rich. Moistened with yogurt or fresh vegetable juice, it makes an excellent exfoliant and pore-tightener for the face.

The flour is easily available in Indian grocery shops; ask for it by its Hindi name, *besan* (pronounced "bay-son").

Five Gram-Flour Beauty Packs

The instructions for each of these are the same. Combine the ingredients, then rub gently on your face. Let the mask tighten on your face for about five minutes. Then rinse with warm water and dab dry with a soft towel.

2 teaspoons gram flour + 1 teaspoon lemon juice + 1½ teaspoons plain yogurt

2 teaspoons gram flour + ½ teaspoon turmeric + 1½ teaspoons table cream

2 teaspoons gram flour + 3 almonds (soaked overnight and finely ground) + 1½ teaspoons cold milk

2 teaspoons gram flour + juice of one tomato

2 teaspoons gram flour + 1 teaspoon grated cucumber + 1 teaspoon clean, filtered water

After rinsing off your gram-flour face pack, treat your face to a rose-petal or lavender sauna (whichever you prefer) to refresh and reopen your pores. It's easy to do: Boil water in a kettle, then switch off the stove and steep 1 cup of the organic flower petals in the water for seven to ten minutes. Now make a tent with the towel to cover both the kettle and your head. Hold your face at a distance of at least 6" above the kettle and steam your face for about ten minutes. Keep your eyes closed during the sauna, and breathe deeply. Make sure the steam from the kettle does not feel uncomfortably hot on your face. Don't dry your skin completely afterward. While still damp, treat your face to a good-quality moisturizer. You'll wear a fresh-from-the-spa glow for hours to come.

This exfoliating, skin-tightening mask is best applied once a week. You can substitute oatmeal or cornmeal flour with the same great results. If your skin is sensitive, use finely ground gram flour and make the mask moister.

teaspoons of clean water to make a runny paste. Stir a few drops of almond or olive oil into the paste, and apply it on your face at night. After a few minutes, rinse it off. Your skin will absorb this lotion with ease, and you'll feel soft and fragrant for less than a dollar. This should make enough almond cream for three nights. Keep the cream refrigerated. You can apply it every night, and you'll soon notice a definite glow to your skin. Make a fresh batch just before you run out so that you'll always have a supply. Take care: Don't use this pack if you are allergic to nuts.

Tea-LC

IF YOU'RE PUTTING THE KETTLE ON, make your teabag do double duty. Once it's out of the cup, let the bag cool down a bit, then place it on the skin under each of your eyes for a soothing touch, enjoying its gentle warmth for a few minutes. The under-eye area is very delicate, so make sure the bag is not uncomfortably hot against your skin. I can never get enough of this Tea-LC.

Refreshing Rice Cleanser

COOKING RICE TONIGHT? Set aside two teaspoons of raw rice grains, and grind them in the blender. The grains will be coarse, but that is as it should be. Make a paste of the rice with a teaspoon of fresh plain yogurt; this will yield just enough pack for one use. Apply the mask to your face for a gentle but effective cleansing experience. The addition of yogurt makes this pack mild enough to be used twice a week.

Silken Milk Moisturizer

POUR TWO TEASPOONFULS of milk into a bowl or saucer. Dip cotton balls in the milk and dab lightly on your face for a soothing, hydrating experience. If you're lactose-intolerant, you can use rice milk or soy milk in the same way. After a few minutes, wash your face with warm water and follow up with a good-quality moisturizing cream. Alternatively, you can hydrate your skin with cotton balls dipped in rosewater. Glycerin and aloe vera gel are also wonderfully soothing to the skin; these can be applied straight out of the bottle, using a light motion of your fingertips. Treat your skin to these rejuvenating ingredients as you putter around in the kitchen, talk on the phone, or watch television.

Lemon Aid

NEXT TIME YOU MAKE LEMONADE, save some of the juice; your skin can use it in many ways. Combine a teaspoon of lemon juice with a few drops of rosewater, and you have a sweet-smelling moisturizer for your hands. Stir together a teaspoon each of cucumber and lemon juice, and you have a good astringent for your skin.

Combined with a teaspoon of granulated sugar, a few drops of lemon juice makes an effective exfoliant for rough areas such as elbows, heels, and knees. Lemon halves, left over from making lemonade, can be rubbed on your elbows and the backs of your hands for an instant refreshing feel.

Mood-Lightening Lavender

MAYBE YOU DON'T USE LAVENDER in everyday cooking. But next time you go to a natural health store, do buy some lavender essential oil. Your senses will love lavender for its lingering, soothing fragrance. Fill a 6-ounce spray bottle with distilled water, and add twelve to fifteen drops of lavender oil. Since essential oil is highly concentrated, just a few drops are enough to infuse the water with a lovely aroma. Spray this refreshing perfume on your skin from time to time. Or spritz your bedsheets with a calming lavender spray to help you sleep well; a good night's rest brings a natural glow to skin. You can make your spray more floral by adding jasmine, ylang-ylang, jojoba, or chamomile essential oils; all of these are soothing and refreshing. I keep cool rosewater in the fridge to mist my skin for both freshness and fragrance. Take care: Before applying a homemade pack or mist, do try it out on a small patch of skin to make sure the blend does not cause irritation.

Sugar Delight

IN THE MOOD for a caramelized apple dessert tonight? Cut back on the brown sugar, and use some of it to slough off old cells from your skin. Simply mix two tablespoons of brown sugar with enough olive oil to make a smooth paste. This will yield just enough mixture for one application. Now add a few drops of vanilla extract for a soft scent, and keep the bowl of paste by your bathtub. Just before your evening bath, rub this mixture on your heels, knees, and elbows. Or you can refrigerate the mix and use it just before your morning shower. The rough texture of the brown sugar, offset by the smoothness of the oil, is perfect for exfoliation. Use this once a week, or whenever possible.

A Pretty, Easy Cleansing Pack

GROUND NUTS, grated orange peel, oatmeal, lentils — these textured foods make excellent exfoliants; rubbed gently on skin, they slough off dead cells and make skin feel wide awake. Whenever you use one of these ingredients in your cooking, set aside one teaspoon of the coarse food and combine it with two teaspoons of almond oil, olive oil, or yogurt to offset the coarseness and make the pack feel soft on your skin. This proportion yields a soft paste, enough for one application. Gently rub the paste into your skin, leave on for five minutes, and rinse it off. Use this pack once a week.

Psst…the Topmost
Secret of Glow-rious Skin

ALL THESE MASKS AND SCRUBS I've suggested will no doubt please your skin. But as you might have noticed, the glow from even the most expensive facial mask doesn't seem to last very long. The reason stares us in the face: Our skin is constantly subjected to so many environmental pollutants and so much stress that it is hard to keep glowing. But — and this is a very happy "but" — you can defeat skin dullness, and quite easily, too! Here's the incredibly simple secret:

Drink water.

I know a woman who drinks about sixteen glasses of water a day. She is forty-five, but her skin looks no more than twenty-five years old. What's more, I've seen her transform within months from a sick, overweight, pale person into a youthful new woman. After removing large stones from her kidney, doctors advised her to drink as much water as she could. She took their advice seriously, and this helped her in more ways than she had imagined. Her digestion improved, the kidney stones never came back, she lost weight without going on a diet, and, as I said, her skin began to shine!

Now, being witness to such an inspiring example I should have found it easy to drink up the recommended eight glasses of water a day. I have to admit that I didn't quite succeed at first. There are days when one simply doesn't feel all that thirsty. It can happen if we're too busy, too stressed, or less thirsty because the weather is cold. When that happens, it's time to pause and get creative.

Discover Delicious Ways to Drink

WITH A LITTLE IMAGINATION, you can treat yourself to some flavorful, energizing, and, yes, beautifying drinks throughout the day. Here are some simple, delicious ideas on how to drink to your health:

Taste Your Water

COULD YOU BE AVOIDING water because it doesn't taste good? If so, invest in a filter or water purifier. It makes a huge difference in the taste. Adding a twist of lime or lemon or a slice of orange or cucumber to the glass helps, too. Another trick I learned: Drink filtered water in a stunning glass; it will taste like champagne! Or buy a water bottle that you really like, and sip water from it through a straw. The fun of sucking on a straw will get you to drink far more than you would from a glass. Besides, you can carry your water bottle anywhere without fear of spills, and the water doesn't get dusty from being in an open container.

Spice Up Your Water

WOULD YOU LIKE TO SPICE UP your drinking water and get plenty of health benefits to boot? Try this: Boil water, then pour it into a thermos. Now add some organic rose petals, whole peppercorns, and crushed cardamom seeds. Close the lid tight. Sip this water all day for a delicious, healing experience. You can also try a hint of cinnamon, a dash of orange peel, or a slice of ginger in your water. Create your own flavorful waters this way, and you'll feel more inspired to drink.

Sip Some Sereni-Tea

NATURAL, DELICATELY FLAVORED, soothing beverages made from petals, roots, seeds, and leaves can change the way you drink.

This world of herbal teas is filled with exciting possibilities. Combine lemon balm with mint, rosemary with lavender, or chamomile with sage. Try fresh organic flower petals such as rose, nasturtium, honeysuckle, or jasmine in your tea. Flavor your tisane with cardamom, cloves, lemon, orange, or ginger. A great cup of herbal tea is ready in no time: Just pour a cup of boiling water over a teaspoon of slightly crushed herbs, and steep for a few minutes to infuse the flavors. You can also make a decoction by simmering the herbs in the water for a few minutes, then straining it into a cup. If you're new to tea-making the herbal way, be patient; it will take you some time to arrive at a favorite flavor. Until then, play with steeping times and quantities. When you have created a recipe you like, give it a name. I call my chamomile and oregano blend "Shan-Tea" (*Shanti* is the Hindi word for peace, and that's just what this tea brings me).

Let Your Creative Juices Flow

I DON'T KNOW ABOUT YOU, but drinking juice is my favorite way to hydrate. When you have no choice but to buy your drink from the office vending machine, choose juice over soda; even artificially flavored juice is better than the completely empty calories you get from a cola.

If you're fortunate enough to work with colleagues who like to exercise and eat healthfully, invite them to start a juicing club. Pool your money to buy a juicing machine (a one-time investment) and juicing ingredients (every week). Set aside some time during the day — say your mid-morning or lunch break — to create juices in your workplace kitchen. Take turns creating juices for the club; this will motivate you to try new flavors and find ways to add extra nutrition.

Here are some of my favorite combinations (these proportions yield one serving of juice):

- 3 strawberries + 10 black grapes + 1 large chunk of fresh pineapple

- 1 peach + 1 pear

- 1 apple + 1 grapefruit

- 1 carrot + 1 beet + 1 tablespoon of wheat grass

- 1/2 cup of blueberries + a handful of pitted cherries

All of these are easy to make, and they're tremendously nourishing. I've arrived at these combinations after trying out different ones, but I'm sure you'll have your own preferences. Be bold: Flirt with new combinations; pack more power into your blends with a few seeds here, some nuts there. Happily for us, nature has endowed our world with a stunning variety of juice-worthy ingredients, such as papaya, watermelon, lemons, oranges, cranberries, kiwi, spinach, and tomatoes. The list is endless, and so are the benefits. Again, think up exciting names for your creations: Berry Refreshing, Mango Melody, whatever!

Just one glass of freshly squeezed fruit or vegetable juice is easy to concoct, loads you with vitamins and other vital nutrients, protects you from disease, boosts digestion, improves circulation, replenishes your energy, cools you down, and tastes delicious.

Cut Back on Caffeine

"AS SOON AS COFFEE is in your stomach, there is a general commotion. Ideas begin to move...similes arise, the paper is covered. Coffee is your ally and writing ceases to be a struggle," said Honoré de Balzac. I'm sure coffee stimulates and energizes all of us, not just writers. But more than three cups a day can spell trouble, because the caffeine then starts forcing the body to flush out water — water the body needs for vital lubrication and digestion. Beyond three cups, the caffeine overload can cause dizziness and heart palpitations. Try this trick the next time you get an urge for caffeine: Postpone drinking it by thirty minutes. Chances are, you'll get busy with something else and forget about it. Or drink a tall glass of water instead. Or try an antioxidant-rich, flavorful herb tea. If nothing works and you really want that coffee now, pour yourself just a quarter cup.

A Word about Inner Radiance

WE'VE ALL COME ACROSS people who look great on the outside, but aren't so likeable up close. Can we call such people beautiful? No, because we find them wanting in what the healers of India call *gunam*, or "good-heartedness."

THOUGHTS FROM SHARMILA AYYENGAR, SOFTWARE PROFESSIONAL, 32

On days when I spend time looking after my skin and hair, my spirits soar. I might be doing something as simple as dabbing my face with cotton dipped in raw milk to give the pores a quick cleanse. Or I could be lightly tapping my face with my fingertips to boost circulation and create a glow. But even these small acts of caring for myself do big things for my self-confidence and my spirits.

On weekends, I treat myself to little face packs and scrubs made at home. An excellent way to moisturize dry skin is this: Bring a quart of whole milk to a boil, then switch off the stove. Let the milk cool to room temperature. Gently scrape away the cream that forms on top of the milk. Apply a small amount of this to your face. After a few minutes, wipe your face with a warm, wet towel. My grandmother used to apply this fresh cream to her skin regularly. If you're so inclined, you can enjoy a nice hot cup of cocoa with the remaining milk. There will be enough left over to share a cup with your whole family.

I come from the southern part of India, where women are known for their long, lustrous hair. Our secret: weekly application of warm castor oil to the scalp, followed by a wash with shikakai powder. The word "shikakai" means "fruit for the hair." Ground and made into a paste with water, shikakai powder lathers moderately and cleans hair beautifully. It is mild and nurturing, and it prevents dandruff. The powder is available at Indian grocery stores. Take care to keep your eyes closed while using shikakai; it is a soap nut and may cause mild irritation of eyes. If that does happen, though, simply wash your eyes thoroughly with cold water and the irritation will subside.

However, it is far easier to judge people and decide that they're "not nice" than to try to walk a few miles in their shoes. The person imbued with true gunam is one who makes that effort. Next time somebody says a harsh word to you or treats you shabbily, don't react immediately. Step out of the scene and watch this person and this crisis from a distance; you're sure to get a new perspective.

Similarly, if you feel the urge to shout at someone, take hold of yourself and try to visualize why this person has done what he or she has done. This will help you understand and forgive.

Over time, this gentle habit of stopping to think, reconsider, and then act will fill you with gunam. Then your mirror will show you a woman as enchanting as a rose, inside and out.

Chapter Summary and Resources

- Believe that you are beautiful, because the Divine resides within each one of us.

- A clean, healthy body is a beautiful body.

- Get rid of hackneyed mind-sets. Think positive thoughts, and you will feel lovely.

- Treat your body to the exquisite pleasure of daily self-massage. Maharishi Ayurveda's Website (www.discover ayurveda.com) has some useful articles on massage and natural skin care.

- Discover the pleasures of a leisurely soak in the bathtub.

- Your kitchen can become the best cosmetics factory in the world. Look up creative homemade cosmetic recipes and ideas on The Dollar Stretcher's Website:

www.stretcher.com. Also check out www.free-beauty-tips.com.

• Drink lots of water and juice to keep your metabolism active and your skin glowing.

• Be good-hearted! You'll glow with inner radiance.

CHAPTER 4

Sanctuary

How to Make Your House a Home

Home is a name, a word, it is a strong one; stronger than magician ever spoke, or spirit ever answered to, in the strongest conjuration.

— CHARLES DICKENS

I feel that when you look at a house, it looks back at you. It's not simply a matter of whether you like a house. It's when the *house* accepts you that it is yours. After having seen and rejected forty-nine beautiful houses in picturesque Colorado Springs, I finally saw my house gazing at me one bright summer afternoon, two years ago.

As I toured the house, every airy nook and sunny corner of it extended a welcome to me. The bay window in the kitchen seemed to say, "Wouldn't I make a bright breakfast nook?" The sunny dining room seemed to be waiting for friends and family, food, conversation, and laughter. The backyard, though bare at the time, felt sweet with the promised fragrance of roses. And was it my imagination, or did the bird on the old oak tree outside the bedroom window actually tweet, "Good to see you! Good to see you!" I felt a strong pang of longing in that moment — a longing to own that smiling house.

Ever since then, I've come to believe that the value of one's living space goes way beyond square-footage and location. You won't find that special quality in the brochures; you'll just feel it, like first love.

Of course, even the most emotionally appealing house remains just that — a house — until you sign the closing papers, move in, and proceed to make it your home.

Welcome Home

YOUR HOME IS A SCRAPBOOK of your life. Its walls, furnishings, artwork, crockery, and books are not lifeless objects. Each one reflects the colors, tastes, smells, textures, and thoughts you like to live with. Your home mirrors your moods and spirits: fresh flowers, soft music, the irresistible aroma of fruit crumble rising from the oven — these are unmistakable signs that you are happy! Your home also reveals your habits and your very nature, telling visitors in an instant whether you are messy or a neatnik, artistic or practical, austere or indulgent, a loner or a lover of company. Quite simply, your house is your canvas; you are free to paint on it the way you like. Isn't that an incredibly empowering and heady thought?

When I say "home," I certainly don't mean just a place you have purchased. I have a friend whose simple touches — fresh blooms, family photographs, well-thumbed books — have transformed a tiny tenement into a cozy cocoon of love. Her secret? She tends her home from the heart. So can you!

Come; make your home a clean, calm, cheerful place to be. I call these the Three Cs of Homemaking.

Home, Clean Home

I ONCE ORDERED an exotic salad at a new restaurant in town. When the waiter brought it, the platter took my breath away with its awesome garnishing. I was so impressed that I took a full minute to admire the presentation. Well, it's a good thing I did, because that's how I spotted a black insect crawling across a dark lettuce leaf. I could feel the juices dry up inside my stomach instantly! It's the same with houses. Even the most exquisite flooring, best artwork, and luxurious furnishings are unattractive if they are dusty and grimy.

So let your first "C" of housekeeping be Clean. If you would rather milk a goat than clean house, here are seven sparkling reasons to make you reach for that sponge. A clean house:

- looks ravishing, even if it is simply and inexpensively decorated;

- heals the mind, because it feels like a temple;

- invites compliments and makes you feel good;

- attracts people;

- repels germs, allergens, and pests;

- saves you time — no more wild hunts for the other sock;

- saves you money — you maintain your belongings better, so they last longer.

If, on the other hand, you're chronically fussy — always brushing imaginary specks of dust from your sofa and microscopic stains from your carpet — take a few quiet moments to remind yourself that:

- this isn't a hotel or a museum — it's your home;

- an ounce of mess isn't worth a ton of stress;

- you'd feel better sharing jokes with your kids than shooing them off carpets;

- maybe you could downsize and de-clutter to reduce the need for constant cleaning.

The bottom line: Somewhere between mess and fuss, there lies a beautifully balanced approach to clean living. A popular kitchen sign summarizes it best: "My home: dirty enough to be happy, and clean enough to be healthy." Stick this sign on your fridge, and read it whenever you're feeling either too messy or too fussy.

Cleaning Is Fun, Naturally

NOW LET'S GET TO THE BRASS TACKS — or, rather, broom straws — of cleaning house. Just as successful cooking begins with the right ingredients, good cleaning begins with good tools.

Let's take a peek beneath your sink. Hmm. I see dishwashing detergent, tile spray, drain opener, furniture polish, carpet stain remover, and several other bottles filled with green and blue liquids. As far as cleaning agents go, you're well stocked.

But let's pause here and picture you spraying that blue liquid from a bottle onto a countertop. Does the spray irritate your throat, hurt your eyes, or make you nauseated? If so, you're not alone. Go to your computer and type "toxins in household cleaners" on Google.com, and you'll get some eye-opening — and, I might add, frightening — information. Here's a small sample of what I found:

PRODUCT	WHAT IT CONTAINS	WHAT IT CAN CAUSE
Bleach	Chlorine fumes	Skin and eye irritation
Carpet cleaner	Perchlorethylene	Anemia, liver and kidney damage
Furniture polish	Nitrobenzene	Skin and lung damage
Bathroom spray	Toxic vapors	Headaches, nausea, shortness of breath, skin rashes, burns, liver

PRODUCT	WHAT IT CAN CAUSE
Bathroom spray	damage, and eye,
(continued)	throat, and lung
	irritation

Yikes! What severe punishments the simple act of cleaning house can perpetrate on an unsuspecting human body! Surf the Internet some more, and you'll find hundreds of horror stories from real people like you and me about how badly their health has suffered from using such harmful cleaning products.

Why suffer when there's a bounty of healthy options to choose from? Dozens upon dozens of pure, natural, nontoxic cleaning agents are sitting right under your nose, waiting for you to notice and use them. Think banana skins (yes, banana skins!), lemon halves, orange peels, rosemary, sage, thyme, eucalyptus, Epsom salt, vegetable oils, essential oils, toothpaste, vinegar, baking soda, and borax. Start looking, and you'll be awestruck at the number of invaluable allies you have in your quest for safe cleaning.

Goodbye Nasty — Hello Natural

IF YOU'RE NEW to natural cleaning, begin with two basic, all-purpose house-cleaning ingredients. You won't find these in the cleaning supplies aisle. Walk across to the salad dressings and baking needs aisles instead! Just pick up:

- baking soda

- distilled white vinegar

End of list. That's all you will need to begin with. Believe it or not, used together these two products can take care of almost all your cleaning needs. They are completely safe, natural, and a breeze to use. Baking soda cleans almost any surface beautifully, while also zapping away odor. Its able assistant, white vinegar, cuts grease, loosens stains, removes rust marks, and refreshes drains.

To use them in combination, mix together:

1 gallon hot water
1/2 cup vinegar
2 tablespoons baking soda

Pour this solution into a spray bottle, shake well, then spritz and wipe. Presto! Your sink smiles, your tiles glow, and your lungs heave a sigh of relief! If you find the smell of vinegar too pungent for your liking — and I know many people do — add ten to fifteen drops of lavender or lemon essential oil to the liquid; you'll be left with a pleasant fragrance in the area after you clean.

Fresh, Clean Ideas for You to Try

WITH THE MONEY YOU SAVE on commercial cleaners (baking soda and a big bottle of vinegar together will cost you less than $5), you can buy eco-friendly cleaning products from a natural health store. Or, more fun, you can create your own cleaning products using inexpensive everyday ingredients. Here are some ideas I've found useful:

Ooh La Loofah!

CLEAN YOUR KITCHEN surfaces with a bath accessory! The humble loofah — which is actually a dried-up vegetable sponge — cleans and wipes spills beautifully, without getting grimy or slimy too quickly. To clean and disinfect your kitchen loofah, simply soak it in a strong solution of Epsom salt and water for 30 to 45 minutes, or until clean. Rinse it out, let it dry, and use it again.

Safely Germ-Free

IN A SPRAY BOTTLE filled with clean water, drizzle a few drops of essential oil, then shake well. Lemon, lavender, clove, eucalyptus,

NATURAL POTPOURRI

Here's an easy recipe for making your own fragrant potpourri:

1 cup lavender

1/3 cup chamomile, peppermint, lemon verbena, or any other dried herbs of your choice

1 tablespoon crushed cinnamon

2 drops rose essential oil

Wearing rubber gloves, mix the lavender, herb, and cinnamon in a medium-sized glass bowl. When the mixture is well blended, add the oil and toss with your gloved hands to coat the mixture evenly. Put an appropriate amount in a bowl or sachet, and store the rest in an airtight glass jar. You can place this potpourri anywhere in the house — in the bedroom, living room, bathroom, or study. Once you discover the joy of creating your own fragrances, you will find a whole new world of scent opening up before you.

pine, spruce, thyme, and grapefruit oils are particularly great for banishing germs. Spray this sweet-smelling mist on any surface to clean and deodorize it.

Another Fragrant Idea

IN A LARGE, clean glass jar, put a handful each of fresh rosemary, sage, and mint leaves. Cover the jar completely with organic apple cider vinegar and close the lid tightly. Let the solution sit undisturbed for one month to six weeks. Then strain the mixture into a spray bottle and use it to disinfect cutting boards, telephones, doorknobs, and other surfaces that attract germs.

Boot Polish? No, Fruit Polish

BANANA SKINS don't always trip you up! They can actually do your tired shoes a great favor. Try it for yourself: Rub a dull leather shoe with the inside of a banana peel, then buff it with a soft flannel cloth to remove banana traces and odor from the surface. Your shoes will shine like new!

Off, Foul Odor!

TAKE A WHIFF. Hmmm, so your carpet smells stale and musty? Don't despair — and, no, don't reach out for that commercial carpet deodorizer. Walk up to your pantry and cut open a few bags of green tea. Sprinkle the tea leaves on your carpet, leave them for fifteen minutes, then vacuum them up. Now sniff all you like; your carpet will smell wonderful. By the way, tea — black or green — is also effective on wooden furniture stains. Dip a cloth in cool tea, and wipe stains off the chair or table.

Don't throw away that used lemon or orange! Drop it in the kitchen sink, add a handful of crushed ice, and run the garbage disposal. This will not only replace the stale-food smell with a fresh citrusy one, but the grinding action will also sharpen the disposal blades.

Another Easy-to-Make Carpet Refresher

POUR TEN TO FIFTEEN DROPS of pine or eucalyptus essential oil into $1/2$ cup of baking soda. Sprinkle the baking soda on a musty carpet. Wait a few minutes, then vacuum it up.

Wide-Awake Windows

POUR 1 CUP OF DISTILLED white vinegar into a 1-quart spray bottle. Top up the bottle with water, add 10 to 12 drops of lemon or orange essential oil to the water-vinegar solution, and shake. Spray the mixture on a dull window and scrub with an old, crumpled newspaper for a good-as-new sparkle.

Lavender Lovers

ADD 10 TO 12 DROPS of lavender essential oil to the rinse cycle of your washing machine for a fresh fragrance. Then fill a spray bottle with water and add 1 drop of lavender essential oil. Spray this fragrant liquid onto clothes before drying or ironing, and you'll never need another fabric softener. Dip a few cotton balls in a mixture of lavender and lemon oils, then tuck the balls into your closet for a soft, sweet smell. Replace the cotton balls once a week, as the oils slowly evaporate.

Bright with Borax

BORAX, OR SODIUM BORATE, is a natural alkaline mineral that you can safely use for cleaning the house. It softens water, deodorizes, disinfects, and repels cockroaches and bugs. Here is one way to use borax for cleaning: Measure 1/2 cup of borax into a bowl, and dip half a lemon into it. Use the lemon to scrub your tiles, basin, and sink.

Don't throw away the leftover borax. Add 1/2 cup of vinegar to it, and dissolve the mixture in warm water to make a loose paste.

Whether you've lived in your house for two years or twenty, revisit your home from time to time as if for the first time. Walk out the door, then reenter, taking in all your observations and feelings:

- How does your home look, feel, and smell?

- Which objects or corners does your eye come to rest on?

- Does something strike you as in need of attention: chipped paint, or a coffee table in need of dusting?

- What adjectives did you think of as you walked in: inviting? calm? vibrant? cheerful? All of these? None of these?

The idea is to keep your home looking and feeling warm and lovely just for you — whether or not you're expecting company.

Apply this paste to areas ridden with mold and mildew, and you'll see quick results.

Paste That Polishes More than Teeth

SQUEEZE SOME WHITE TOOTHPASTE into a small bowl, and dilute it with warm water just like you would paint. Now dip an old toothbrush in the paste, and scrub your silver with it. You'll be rewarded with a rich sparkle.

Mayo Magic

IS YOUR WOODEN DINING table looking dull? Dip a soft cloth in leftover mayonnaise, and rub the table with it; you'll be surprised at the sheen. Try this mayo treatment on wooden chairs and staircase railings, too. To make sure your surfaces aren't left greasy or messy with the mayo, simply run a clean cloth over the surface to add luster and remove all traces of mayo.

THESE ARE JUST A FEW IDEAS; dozens more easy and exciting ones are waiting for you to discover them. So start a journal of safe cleaning tips. Fill it with ideas and recipes from friends who use natural ingredients, or try your own. You'll be amazed at the fresh possibilities that open up. Take care: Essential oils can burn skin upon direct contact, and ammonia reacts strongly with bleach to give off dangerous fumes. So don't experiment with ingredients without reading up on their properties.

Now that you've tucked the brooms back in the cupboard and put out the sponges — and loofah — to dry, treat yourself to a refreshing drink of juice or herbal tea. As you relax, take in the calm environment of your home, letting it restore and energize you once again.

Home-Calming

"CALM. *Adjective*. Peaceful and quiet; without hurried movement, anxiety, or noise."[1] That is how the Cambridge online dictionary defines "calm." Is your home a calm, peaceful place? Of course, if you have a house full of little children you might laugh at the question. But when I say calm, I'm not referring to an absence of sound; I mean absence of *noise*. Yes, there is a subtle difference.

Sound in itself can be a source of pleasure and restfulness. For example:

- Peppers sizzling in a pan
- Children laughing
- Bees humming
- Birds singing
- Wind chimes jingling
- A brook running
- A musician playing a melody

It is when sound becomes noise — disturbing, jarring sound — that it agitates the mind and makes the heart restless. Not surprisingly, the word "noise" has its origin in the Latin word "nausea," which means "sickness." Noise can be as quiet as the constant drip-drip of a leaky tap, or as loud as a high-decibel shouting match between husband and wife. In a different but equally important sense, clutter and dirt are visual "noise."

I'll tell you what. No matter how "noisy" your life seems right now, you can start living more calmly and happily in one month's time. What's more, you can do it by devoting just five to ten minutes a day to removing the clutter from your life. And I mean real, physical clutter.

Simplify!

HERE ARE SOME TRUTHS about clutter:

- Clutter grows.

- Clutter occupies prime real estate, costing you money.

- Clutter reflects poor habits and an indecisive state of mind.

- Clutter irritates the senses and disturbs the mind. And when you are unsettled in your mind, you argue more, fret more, stress more. All of which increases the "noise" around you.

- Therefore, clutter deserves to go.

But before you pick up the first piece of paper for junking or filing, recognize the mindsets that commonly block our path to clutter-free living.

Cluttered thinking: "I might just need this magazine article/ CD/ video cassette someday."

Clear thinking: "I haven't used this for a long time, and I don't need this right now or in the near future. Let me sell it or give it away. I can always buy another one if need be."

So clip out the article, file it away, and throw out the magazine. Record all your favorite songs on a handful of CDs and give away the rest. If you really cannot part with the videocassette of *Casablanca*, make a deal with yourself: The cassette stays if you give away one other thing you can afford to part with.

Cluttered thinking: "I'll clear that closet tomorrow."

Clear thinking: "Who knows, I might be even busier or more tired tomorrow? Better than nothing, I'll sort out just ten items of clothing while I have a few minutes."

Sort clothes into these categories:

- To Repair

- To Return or Exchange

- To Refresh (wash/dry-clean/iron/starch)

- To Give Away

- To Wear

Cluttered thinking: "I can't do anything about this stuff until I have shopped for the right shelves and containers to put it in."

Clear thinking: "I might not have time to go container shopping soon. Until then, why not junk, sell, or give away things I don't need? That way, I'll save money on buying too many containers — which could become part of the clutter, too!"

Cluttered thinking: "I can't possibly part with those photos/clothes/greeting cards; they bring back so many memories..."

Clear Thinking: "Of course I can't junk all those memories, but surely I can select the best ones and discard the rest. Instead of

SOFTEN YOUR SURROUNDINGS

Situation: You spend most of your waking day inside an office where the harsh environment — steel, glass, plastic, cables, papers — makes you feel overloaded and overwhelmed.

Solution: Say the word "soft." Say it out out loud. Taste it on your tongue. Delicious, isn't it?

Think of the soft sights, sounds, and textures you love. Yielding chenille pillows. Delicate rosebuds. Mellow music. Simply thinking of these things can make you feel so good! Imagine being suffused with such soft sensations when you come home.

Maybe you can't get rid of all that steel, glass, and plastic, but if you cushion it with some softness you'll create a home that is synonymous with serenity.

all the drawings my son ever made, I'll keep only the first one and two others that are truly appealing. All those trunks filled with baby clothes... Let's be realistic: My daughters are now grown up, and other children can make good use of those lovingly preserved garments. I'll keep just a few, and give the rest away."

Don't you feel better — more sorted out — just reading these ideas? Follow them, and you'll feel as if you've thrown open your windows and your lungs to a fresh blast of air. And you won't be wrong, either, because ancient wisdom from India and China says that removing clutter increases essential energy, which we know today as *chi, qui, prana,* or life-force.

How to Surround Yourself with Serenity

AS CLUTTER MAKES A SLOW but steady exit from your home, think of ways to enhance your newfound sense of calm by harnessing elements such as color and nature.

Harmonize with Color

ARE YOU EASILY RUFFLED? Do you find it difficult to sleep? Are you possessive, jealous, ambitious? If so, take a look at the colors in your house. Too much color or too many busy patterns — stripes, checks, dots — can create visual noise. That is why you'll never find a monastery decorated in psychedelic colors. Try to bring cool, soothing colors such as surf-white, earth-green, and sky-blue into your life. Paint a bathroom wall a lovely pastel blue. Indulge in all-white bed linen — with white sheets, white pillows, and a white comforter. Replace those hot-colored cushions with various shades of green; your living room will feel like a quiet forest.

If, on the other hand, you're lethargic, dull, and prone to depression, a splash of rose-red or sunrise-yellow can actually be soothing to your soul. Paint one wall of your dining room a brilliant red; used in small bursts, red is known to stoke the appetite. Frame yellow-orange pictures in your living room. Buy a sprightly pink lamp!

Relax with Art and Literature

CREATE OR BUY ART with a spiritual theme. Or frame quotations and poems that make you feel peaceful. I used to have a fear of dark rooms, until my mother gave me a poster that said: "Sleep in peace, God is awake."

Create a cozy "book-nook" in your home — it could be a large shelf full of your favorite books, or even a few of your best-loved bedside volumes. The printed word can be a great source of companionship, inspiration, and good cheer. Besides, books stacked on a shelf, piled up in a basket, or strewn across a coffee table bring that irresistible "stay-on-and-make-yourself-at-home" look to the barest of spaces. If you cannot afford to buy all the books you love — and many of us cannot — borrow from your local public library. Keep some fine books by your bedside, but don't read them too close to bedtime. Ancient Ayurvedic healers of India believed in moving away from all kinds of sensory stimulation at night. I've found this to be valuable advice. Even if a book leaves you with pleasant thoughts, they are still thoughts; what you really need is to detach yourself from them at bedtime. So a few minutes before I close my eyes, I close my book and put it away. Then I breathe slowly and deeply until sleep steals in.

Unwind with Sound

HAVE YOU SPENT A DAY in the woods, sitting by a brook and listening to the music of flowing water? How healing that sound is! Simulate the rhythm of the brook in your home: Bring home a water fountain. Dim the lights, put your feet up, and enjoy the natural music of water from time to time. I have an audiotape with nothing on it but the sound of falling rain. Listening to it brings back memories of my childhood days in the city of Delhi, when we would get soaked to the skin and come home to a treat of hot onion fritters and lots of spiced, milky tea. You might enjoy ocean sounds or wind blowing in the desert. Try this sound therapy when you're stressed; you'll feel supremely serene.

Heal with Scent

FOR CENTURIES, scent has been used to heal the senses. Today it is an established fact that some scents, such as lavender, increase the alpha brain waves associated with relaxation. To dissolve anxiety, place a few drops each of ylang-ylang and jasmine in a vaporizer to scent your room. Fill pretty spray bottles with fragrances of your choice: geranium promotes peace, and rose is excellent for after-dinner relaxation. Sniff the oils straight from the bottles or dab some oil on a clean handkerchief. Invite scent into your home with natural scented candles, incense, diffusers, and freshly moistened potpourri — taking care not to overwhelm yourself with the smells, of course!

House Cheerful

CHEER, THE THIRD "C" in my list of homemaking basics, is a heartwarming word. Think cheer, and what are the first images that float into your mind? To me, a cheerful home is not only exuberant with color and texture, but also aglow with light and laughter.

Light Beautiful

THERE'S A BEAUTIFUL Pakistani made-for-television miniseries called *Dhoop Kinare*, which means "On the shore of sunlight." In the story, one of the characters says to her friend, "A little darkness cannot dim a lot of light. But a little light can drive away a lot of darkness." Those words touched me deeply when I heard them, and while they were said in a more metaphorical way, I think they are true in the physical sense, too.

Light is indeed intimately linked to our emotions. In fact researchers have found that sunshine fills you with energy, boosts your metabolism, regulates your sleep-wake cycle, and improves your mood (have you ever felt like dancing on a dull, cloudy day?).

While you cannot do much about the color of the sky on a given morning, you can certainly invite cheerful light inside your home — even if you have a cold, north-facing bedroom or a home with many dark corners. Here are some easy ways to do this:

• Undress your windows! Open them up and discard the drapes. Shop for simple Venetian blinds or sheer white curtains. Try bamboo and canvas — so elegant in their simplicity.

• Invest in a skylight or two. It's truly worth the money if your room craves sunlight.

• If a room — such as a basement — is really beyond the reach of natural light, perk it up with a bright indoor light. This doesn't have to mean a trip to Pier 1 Imports. Why not create your own lamps? Ever since I made a lamp out of an old coffee can, I've been hooked. A trip to your local hardware store should provide you with a lamp-making kit — containing a cord with a switch, a threaded rod, a candelabra socket, a candle cover, a chandelier bulb, and simple instructions on how to put them all together. Use your imagination to come up with ideas for the base and the shade. Basically, anything with a solid base, such as bottles, jars, kettles, or books can work as a lamp base. Brighten up a boring lampshade with a touch of fabric paint, a trimming of coordinating fabric, or glued-on beads and buttons. You can find dozens of ideas for creating and decorating your own lamps and shades on the website www.diy.net.

If you're new to the world of indoor lighting, don't get swamped by the vocabulary — uplights and downlights, incandescents and fluorescents. Think from instinct. Would this corner feel cozy washed in a pool of light? Or would the room look bigger and brighter with a circle of light on the ceiling? Then, when you're sure you know where you would like the light to fall, you'll be able to ask the right questions at the store and get just what you want.

A row of candles, to me, is like a row of mini-suns. Anywhere you light a candle, you create a happy glow. Rub some olive oil or any other cooking oil on a fresh green apple to give it a sheen, then core it and tuck a bright red candle inside. Light a huge chandelier with real candles. Or buy a country-style sconce for your most beautiful candle, and create instant magic for your wall. Take care: Never leave a burning candle unattended.

Use your imagination to think of other ways to make your home brighter: Light a cozy fire; paint your walls a vivid yellow to simulate sunshine; paint your ceilings a light color to reflect whatever light is available.

The sunniest touch in a home is laughter. Did you know that an average person laughs thirteen times a day? Don't be an average person! Find time for humor in your life. Read up on jokes; collect them and share them with your family and friends. You'll feel like new. Seriously!

The Little Things That Add Big Cheer

OF COURSE, if your family is warm and friendly, you can make your home feel like July even in January. But in addition to the human touch, some sweet and simple decorations will also add to the make-yourself-at-home feel of your place.

Brighten up with Baskets

STEEL CONTAINERS are sturdy, no doubt, and glass looks good. But nothing beats the warmth and cheer of a handmade basket. You can store and display almost anything in baskets: magazines, crayons, towels, linen, laundry, buttons, flowers, fruits, popcorn, bread, cosmetics, shoes, letters — the list is endless. Imagine thirsty white towels piled inside a roomy wicker basket, picnic snacks in a casual basket against a bright red-and-white tablecloth, or a happy collection of herb pots inside a roomy basket. Yes, a basket is beauty at its simplest and most charming.

Play with Pictures

A SWEET MEMORY is instant warmth; a collection of memories is a bouquet of joy. One of my friends chose twelve of her favorite family photos, took them to a copy shop, and had them blown up and printed onto a New Year calendar. Each time her family turns the page to a new month, they take a fresh trip down memory lane. What a wonderful idea! Another person I know had a bunch of baby pictures of herself and her husband blown up and hung on a wall. It is great for their children to see what their parents looked like as kids, and it reminds the parents of a happy, simple time in their lives. I once clipped my favorite family photographs onto a lampshade with clothespins. The idea was an instant hit, and the photos provided just the right atmosphere for an evening of intimate conversation. Another lovely idea: Cover your dining table with fun family photos, and lay a sheer fabric or a sheet of glass over them.

Invite Nature In

WE ALL LOVE TO DECORATE with paintings, artifacts, lamps, and such. You can find most of these just a short drive away, at your nearest antique store or shopping mall. But some of the best, most satisfying home décor items are available to you entirely free of cost. You'll find them while strolling by a river, walking through the woods, or right there in your backyard. Here are some simple, inspiring ideas:

Pretty in Pink: Nature has painted her berries, radishes, rhubarb, and potatoes in all shades of pink. Why hide these beauties in the fridge or in dark cupboards? Bring them out, place them in glass jars or on plates, and enjoy them in their full glory. The queen of the pink family is, of course, the lovely rose. And don't forget the dainty delphinium.

Yo! Yellow: The yellow family, like so many other color families, is a jolly big one. You're looking at hues like sunflower yellow, butter yellow, lemon, mimosa, and many others. What's more, each shade plays up differently against different surfaces; try your favorite yellow on a fabric, a sheet of paper, a book jacket, a piece of paper, against a wall. Each time, you'll find the tone changing from simply yellow to orangish, reddish, mustardish, greenish, warm, muted, bright, or flat. But don't limit yourself to buying paint or wallpaper. Think sunshine streaming in through windows, sunflowers and daffodils nodding in vases, fresh-cut lemons and healthy bananas on your table, corn and yellow peppers in ceramic bowls.

Clean Green: What a choice of materials you have: leaves, grass, seaweed, apples, vegetables, herbs, cardamom. Bring home the restfulness of green with any or all of these eye-pleasing plants. You might make a bouquet of fresh herbs in a colorful cup, place a few pods of cardamom in a silver bowl, or build a mini-mountain of fresh green apples, waiting to be sliced for a juicy pie.

Virginal White: White is, well, white, right? Not really. An Indian poet spoke of four tones of white: the greeny-white of sea foam, the blue-white of clouds, the yellow-white of early sunshine, and the silver-white of sand. In your home, the varied tones of white can create magic, using such simple things as seashells, snowflakes, eggs, garlic pods, rice, and gardenia flowers. Especially on days when you are longing for some calm, set out these ingredients in simple bowls and jars to give your eyes — and through them, your heart — a sense of serenity.

Warm Brown and Rich Red: Long ago, I read a sentence that stuck in my mind: "It rained, and the mud turned the color of chocolate-cake batter." Nature is so rich with earthy browns: pinecones, jute, seeds, nuts, chilies, terra-cotta, cinnamon sticks, driftwood, barks. But on its own, brown can be dull and depressing; combine it, as nature does, with bright reds and yellows. Think red roses, peppers, tomatoes, red cabbage, cranberries, strawberries, raspberries, or cherries. Propped against a soothing white background, these simple combinations can make a real splash. Then there are the honeyed brown tones of natural fibers. Try roll-up blinds, trays, screens, and wind chimes made of bamboo; this earth-friendly fiber is great-looking, trendy, and versatile. Bring home rugs, carpets, and even wall-coverings made from sisal, another durable and lovely natural fiber whose warm beige, golden wheat, and coconut shades are gaining tremendous popularity. Learn how you can use other eco-friendly fibers such as coir, jute, sea grass, and mountain grass to decorate your home without allergens and chemicals.

Give Your Guest Room the Personal Touch

MAKE YOUR GUESTS FEEL snug-as-a-bug-in-a-rug. You don't have to decorate your guest room expensively; just a few thoughtful touches will show that you care. Here are some reminders:

- Supply extra blankets, because people have different temperature preferences.

- Make sure the guest room, the bathroom, and the hall to the bathroom have nightlights so that guests can find their way around easily.

- Provide warm touches, such as fresh flowers, new magazines, good books, candles, and an array of natural soaps and lotions.

If you get unexpected visitors, don't worry. As long as you like your visitors, you can relax — and so can your guests. In India, the Hindi word for guest is *atithi,* which means "without a date" — in other words, a person who could drop in anytime, unannounced. And *atithi satkar,* or "making a guest feel welcome," is a venerable tradition. That is why, if you visit an Indian family, you shouldn't be surprised if you are asked "tea, or something cold?" so many times that you have to give in!

Create and Reinvent Often

I DON'T KNOW about you, but I cannot bear to be surrounded by never-changing arrangements and objects in my house. So, whenever possible, I move a painting here, a vase there — and completely redecorate a wall someplace else. But even if you belong to the once-and-forever school of thought, do give these fun, random ideas a try some time:

- Scout yard sales for exciting bargain buys, such as beads, lace, ribbon, old signs, pretty pebbles and shells, old art supplies, trunks, jugs, and interesting bottles. But don't buy things totally on impulse. Take a moment to visualize where and how you can use that "terrific find" in you house. If ideas don't come, the find might not be so terrific after all.

- Gather a few picnic baskets, stack them up, and — presto! You have a coffee table! Stack another one on top, and you've got an end table. To give your table stability, and your home a storage solution, fill the baskets with books, magazines, photo albums, or any other objects that need a home.

- Are you scrambling for a centerpiece for dinner guests? Don't think large or expensive. Create enchantment with blue glass bottles lined up in a row on the table. Slip single daisies in each one. Or paint empty soup cans in cheerful colors and use them to display country-style bouquets.

- Show off your sink! Showcase cleaning products — such as baking soda and vinegar — in pretty bottles. Throw out that frayed, smelly dishcloth, and replace it with a fresh one. Clean out your garbage disposal. Tuck wildflowers in tiny bottles around the area. Wish you were on vacation? Create a beachy look at dinner tonight by placing candles and shells in sand-filled galvanized pails or old milk cans on the table. Place wildflowers and stones around the dinner plates for a seaside feel. Take care: Make sure the candles are firmly in place, and never leave burning candles unattended.

- It's summertime, and the weather is gorgeous. Bring out your prettiest table napkins and towels, and show them off on a clothesline! Add interest to the proceedings with bunches of flowers clipped together on the line.

- Ring in the old! Rescue old dressers, mirrors, and chairs from yard sales. Give them a fresh coat of paint and a new lease on life. Then place old photographs in old frames against old mirrors around these finds, and create the perfect country look at very little expense.

- A table napkin is just a square piece of cloth, right? Look again! With a few strokes of fabric paint or a pen, you can make your napkins the talk of the table. Simply write your favorite food quotations on them. My own favorite is the old saying, "Never trust a thin cook"!

I will leave you to enjoy your clean, calm, cheerful home with this traditional Irish blessing:

May you always have walls for the winds, a roof for the rain, tea beside the fire, laughter to cheer you, those you love near you, and all your heart might desire.

Chapter Summary and Resources

- Your home is your personal sanctuary. Choose it with care.

- The three Cs of homemaking are cleanliness, calm, and cheer. Here are two inspiring books about the home: *The Natural House*, by Daniel D. Chiras (Chelsea Green Publishing, 2000), and *A Room of Her Own: Women's Personal Spaces*, by Chris Casson Madden (Clarkson Potter, 1997).

- Rid your home of toxic commercial cleaning products. Make safe cleaning solutions yourself, or buy them at a natural products store. Read up on natural alternatives for clean living so that you can enjoy their benefits safely. I recommend *Organic Style* magazine (www.organicstyle.com), a gold mine of information on natural living. Another wonderful resource is *Natural Home Magazine* (www.naturalhomemagazine.com). As for

THOUGHTS FROM JOANN PINTO,

DOLL MAKER, 47

I think that, just as a river wends its way to the ocean, we also move toward a place where we truly feel "at home" at last.

Until a few years ago, my husband and I were caught up in the pace of life in California. We didn't realize how fast we were riding the roller coaster until we faced a personal crisis. That event forced us to stop and ask some basic questions: "Where are we heading?" "What do we really want to do?" And the answer came spontaneously: We needed a change of environment — an unhurried, healing place where we could be whole again.

So my husband gave up his thriving medical practice, I gave up my job, and we moved to the forests of Colorado. Brick by loving brick, we built ourselves a house that has become a healing sanctuary for all our needs. Physically, emotionally, spiritually, this is where I want to be. It is a sanctuary in the true sense of the word.

I now make dolls that depict simple life truths: love, blessings, joy. They help me heal, and I know they help others heal, too. My doll-making has connected me to hundreds of people across the country; I attend lectures, workshops, and exhibitions, meeting like-minded women and enjoying my life to the fullest.

People are always struck when I tell them about our drastic career switch and the decision to move from a pulsating city to a home in the wilderness. But I strongly feel that when you decide from the heart, all the positive forces of the universe come together to back you in your effort. They did so for me. That is why I have come home.

the Internet, there is so much useful information out there that all you have to do is type "nontoxic house-cleaning ideas" on the powerful search engine Google.com, and you'll be presented with hundreds of surf-worthy sites.

• A clutter-free home is a calm home. Hundreds of books have been written on the subject of clearing clutter from your life. Browse some and select ones that you feel will address your own problem points. The Internet is also a rich resource for ideas on reducing clutter.

• Harness color, light, and texture to create a bright, joyful home. For ideas, look up Websites such as Home and Garden Television's www.hgtv.com and *Ladies' Home Journal's* site, www.lhj.com.

• Simple things, such as baskets, pictures, and flowers can make your home sing with warmth.

• Let your home be an invitation for guests to feel comfortable and welcome.

• Be creative! Reinvent your home with fun touches every now and then.

• Get inspiration from friends. Go shopping with those who have a good sense of style. Meet more people. The more homes you see, the more ideas you'll get.

• Watch home-decorating shows on television. I enjoy "Decorating Cents," "Flea Market Finds," and "Gardening By the Yard" on Home and Garden Television. Also check out "Home Matters" on the Discovery channel.

- Learn about decorating from everything around you. Read books and magazines — an evergreen resource for ideas. Take a course in home decorating. Look on the Internet for ideas. Go out: Look at how nature combines her colors and frames her pictures; you're sure to come back inspired.

CHAPTER 5

Love

How to Nurture Your Relationships

Love is life. All, everything that I understand,
I understand only because I love.
Everything is, everything exists, only because I love.

— LEO TOLSTOY

*A*h! The cozy world of love. Whispered words, stolen kisses, moonlit walks, love notes, phone calls, warm hugs, laughter...Why do these joys seem like luxuries today? Why is it that we're somehow missing deep emotional contentment in our lives? Do you often wonder about this and feel wistful? If so, I've got some cheering news: You can put the magic back in your relationships! Yes, you can be a loving spouse, a solid friend, a caring mom, and a kind colleague — without quitting your job or compromising on your commitments. All you need is a deep desire to make your heart a happier, more loving place. Ready to begin? Here's the first step:

Think about the Word "Connection"

CELL PHONE, PAGER, the World Wide Web — thanks to technology, we're better "connected" than ever before. But then, aren't these tools also slowly distancing us from real, in-person communication? Haven't all those voice-mails and e-mails almost replaced the touch of a hand, a smile, a hug?

No, I'm not suggesting that you toss your cell phone, log off your computer forever, and go back to the Middle Ages. But, yes, you can use technology selectively so that it doesn't become an invasive, all-pervasive influence in your life. How? Just press a few "off" buttons from time to time.

At your first opportunity today, disconnect the phone, switch off the computer, turn off the television, and put away any newspapers or magazines you've been reading. Basically, filter out the "noise" from all artificial tools of communication until you experience nothing but your five senses. You are now tuned in to the real world as it hums around you, complete with sight, sound, and touch:

- Your eyes, no longer distracted by the computer screen or TV, are able to notice other people.

- Your ears, freed from the cell phone, are able to hear people's voices — up close and personal.

- Your hands, removed from the mouse, the remote control, or the receiver, are free to hold other people's hands. Your senses come alive to the intimate beauty of human touch.

Most importantly, your mind, temporarily released from the fully wired, hyperefficient world, has the opportunity to relate to real human beings. You listen instead of just hearing, you observe instead of just looking, and you feel instead of just touching.

But before you set out to connect with others, let me remind you of a standard airline safety instruction: "First put on your own oxygen mask; only then try to help a fellow passenger." I think the logic applies equally to life; you cannot make other people happy if you are feeling overdrawn and drained from within. So, for your loved ones' sake, be good to yourself! Find ways to be happy so that you can make them happy. A pleasant assignment, isn't it? Come, let me show you some easy ways to gladden your heart,

THE BEST THINGS
ANYONE EVER SAID ABOUT LOVE

Love is an irresistible desire to be irresistibly desired.

— Robert Frost

Love is the wisdom of the fool and the folly of the wise.

— Samuel Johnson

Love gives naught but itself and takes naught but from itself. Love possesses not nor would it be possessed; For love is sufficient unto love.

— Kahlil Gibran

Love must be as much a light as a flame.

—Henry David Thoreau

To love someone is to wish him life.

—Chinese Proverb

Love conquers everything [Amor vincit omnia]: let us, too, yield to love.

—Virgil

Shall I compare thee to a summer's day? Thou art more lovely and more temperate: Rough winds do shake the darling buds of May, and summer's lease hath all too short a date.

— William Shakespeare

If you judge people, you have no time to love them.

— Mother Teresa

Love is like a butterfly: hold it too tightly and you'll crush it, hold it too loosely, and it will fly away.

— Unknown

brighten your spirits, and generally make you a pleasant person to be around.

Self-Nurturing Made Simple

HAVING COME FROM THE DRY, hot plains of India, I found the fall season in the U.S. incredibly beautiful. The first year of our stay in America, my husband and I couldn't take enough photographs of those mountains ablaze with bright orange-yellow-red trees in the crisp October air.

As winter crept in, we promised that next fall we'd capture time-lapse pictures of maple leaves changing color. We dreamed of taking the famous train trip between Durango and Telluride. But that didn't quite happen; we got busy with our jobs, and our son got caught up in school. For three years, October came and went, but we were too busy to take a single weekend off.

So we did the next best thing: We combined our grocery-shopping and errand-running with short drives around the neighborhood. Watching the sun's fading light catch the gorgeous roadside trees wasn't the same as reveling in a valley of color, but it was something — and we'll cherish the memories of those evenings forever.

Looking after your own health and well-being is somewhat like that. You can keep postponing the big things — checking into a spa, taking an RV trip to Alaska, joining a meditation class — "until there's enough time and money." Or you can give yourself some lovely little pleasures right here, right now.

Here's my list of just-for-you gifts that you can squeeze into an ordinary day.

A soothing cup of herbal tea: This is a great way to find calm without caffeine, chemicals, or calories. Besides, the very act of slowly sipping tea is a welcome respite from the day's hurried pace. I especially love the flavor and fragrance of sweet basil, lemon balm, and chamomile, but of course there are endless other combinations waiting to be tried and enjoyed. Here's a must-try iced-tea recipe for times when you're longing for a soothing sip:

HERBAL ICED TEA

4 cups water
1 chamomile tea bag
1 lavender tea bag
zest of one orange or lemon
fresh ginger root, peeled and sliced
honey to taste

Boil the ingredients together, then cover and simmer for about ten minutes. Remove the pan from the heat and chill the brew for at least eight hours. Pour into a tall glass filled with crushed ice, and enjoy this great antidote to stress.

A pore-awakening face pack: Does your skin sometimes feel so dull and grimy that you begin to sulk? Take a few minutes to rub a gentle granular pack on your face. As the dead cells fall off, both your skin and your spirits will wake up. Here's an easy pack to try: Mix one tablespoon of oatmeal with one tablespoon of plain yogurt. Apply the mixture gently to your face, then wash it off with tepid water after a few minutes. Afterward, you'll be smiling at everyone! (For other easy-to-make natural face-pack recipes, turn to chapter 3.)

A walk in the park or a stroll on the sidewalk: If you spend most of your waking hours confined to an office, a short reprieve from your surroundings can work wonders for your spirits. In the first few minutes of your lunch hour, amble out to take in the simple sights and sounds of life — trees swaying,

I remember the day when I sprang out of bed, rushed to my office, and opened my e-mail, expecting to find an urgent communication I had been waiting for. Instead, I found a chain letter. My first thought was to sue the sender. Then I read the e-mail. Here is what it said:

A philosophy professor is teaching his class. He has brought with him an empty glass jar, some rocks, some pebbles, and a box of sand. Wordlessly, he fills up the jar with the rocks, and asks his students if the jar is full. They agree that it is.

Next, he adds the pebbles to the rocks in the jar. As expected, the pebbles settle into the spaces between the rocks. Then he pours the sand into the jar, and immediately, the sand covers everything else.

"Now," says the professor, "Think of this jar as your life. The rocks are the important things — your family, your partner, your health, your children — anything that is so important to you that if it were lost, you would be nearly destroyed. The pebbles are the other things that matter, like your job, your house, your car. The sand is everything else: the small stuff.

"If you put the sand into the jar first, you won't be able to fit the pebbles or rocks in. The same goes for your life. If you spend all your energy and time on the small stuff, you will never have room for the things that are important to you. Pay attention to the things that are critical to your happiness: Play with your children, take time to call a friend, go out dancing with your spouse.

"There will always be time to clean the house, pay the bills and fix the garbage disposal. Take care of the big rocks first — the things that really matter. Set your priorities. The rest is just sand."

Few stories have ever touched me the way this one did. The first thing I did after reading it was to call home and tell my son I was sorry I had left without giving him a hug. Then I took half the day off and spent it with my family — at a carnival.

children playing, people walking, clouds floating by. You'll return to work feeling brighter.

A date with your car. This might sound silly, but I have an intimate relationship with my car; it is my own private space for listening to music, singing for my own pleasure, or just enjoying the silence. On days when I can afford the time, I cruise down un-crowded winding lanes, relishing the feel of the road beneath the wheels and admiring the trees that stand like bouquets along the way.

Dancing to your favorite music. Studies show that harmonious sound releases feel-good hormones, called endorphins, in the brain. But you don't need a scientist to tell you that; I'm sure your heart's response to a good melody has told you on many occasions. In fact, if you think back to all the good times you've had, I'm sure you'll realize that music played a part in making them special. So dim the lights (bright lights are jarring to the senses), put on your favorite CD, and twist, jive, or gently sway to the cadence — or just sit and let the melody carry you away.

Lying on your back, watching the night sky. This is as close as it gets to perfection for me: a pillow of green grass, a clear night filled with stars, and a silence in which I can hear myself think.

Slipping into your softest pajamas and curling up with a good book. Need I say more?

I INVITE YOU TO make a list of your own simple pleasures. Don't worry that such a list is "not for you" because you'll never have time. Remember the beautiful words of writer Richard Bach in his book *Illusions:* "We are never given a wish without also being given the power to fulfill it."[1] Yes, you have the power to free up time for yourself. Come on, exercise that power. Press that "off" button, and watch the seconds and minutes add up for you to enjoy. Here are some ways to take a break from technology and connect with yourself:

- Keep the cell phone off while you drive. This will not only help avoid collisions, but it will allow you to sing to yourself or spend time recalling a special moment you shared with your family or friends. It is also a great time to get creative and think of special things you can do for yourself and others.

- Every day, take a short respite from the computer. Set aside a definite time to do this — say, a few minutes during the 4:00 coffee break. Use that time to write yourself a note, a story, or a poem. Or spend that time rubbing lotion on your fingers, massaging your wrists, or gently pressing your tired knuckles. That way, you'll give something back to the hands that make it possible for you to do so many wonderful things.

- Prepare a "vacation-mail" and send it as an auto-respond copy to all your friends who have sent you e-mail. Let it read thus: "I'm taking a day off from the Internet to do some feel-good things for myself. Your e-mail is special to me, and I promise to reply to you tomorrow." Your message might actually inspire the sender of the e-mail to do the same thing for herself!

Now imagine taking such healing breaks not once a day, but for a whole luscious day! Wondering when you'll ever find that kind of time? Well, how about this coming Sunday?

Have a Me Day

I HAVE A POLICY: On Sundays, I don't allow myself to come within five hundred yards of the computer; the phone goes on voice mail; and the cell phone gets to snooze in my purse all day.

It works fine because, fortunately, there's no danger of missing out on business calls or office work on Sundays. My friends know how I am about Sundays, and they respect my need for solitude. This soothing Sunday routine means a lot to me. It's officially Me Day, and it's wonderful to enjoy fifty-two such days a year — days in which I can be as lazy or as active as I want to be.

Give yourself a Me-Day. I promise you'll emerge from it feeling your nurturing best. Even if you don't consciously set out to pamper yourself, a Me Day can be made special just by reveling in the restorative power of solitude. Do something as "wasteful" as staying in bed all day with a trashy novel, or as "sinful" as spending the day watching television with lots of chocolate, ice cream, and popcorn. As long as it makes you feel good, do exactly as you please.

Here's one of the many ways to orchestrate your Me Day: The night before, try to get to sleep early —10:00 p.m. at the latest — so that you'll wake up feeling rested and ready to greet the morning light. As you open your eyes, revel in the thought that a brand-new gift of a day awaits you — ready to be unwrapped layer by beautiful layer. Step out on your terrace, patio, or balcony and feel the early sunshine and the fresh morning air on your face.

Do plan some healing activities for the day, but don't pressure yourself to fulfill them. The idea is to relax in the true sense of the word. Have a luxurious soak in the bathtub, cook a light meal, take an afternoon nap, enjoy your tea out in the deck or in your favorite nook at home — and in the evening, take some time to plan breakfast and set out your clothes for the next morning.

But, as I said before, this is just one of the many healing ways to script your day. Think of the things you would most like to do today. If you're not sure, try completing this sentence: "My idea of a perfect self-nurturing day is…" I'm sure this enjoyable exercise will uncork your imagination! Here are some more Me Day ideas for you to pick from:

Spend an afternoon in a park. Watch ducks floating in the pond and cuddly dogs trotting alongside their masters; feel the gentle ripple of the breeze in your hair; see the sunshine filtering through leaves. If the mood hits you, whoosh down a slide or enjoy a swing, write a poem under a shady tree, or lie down on a bench and dream.

Go for a walk by yourself at the beach. If you live near the ocean, do it just to connect with the water and rub your feet in the sand; it's a wonderfully natural way to rid your feet of calluses and heal your mind.

Check into a hotel or spa for the day. Pamper yourself with a rejuvenating treatment. Or just lie in the comfort of your hotel bed, enjoying the temporary disconnection from your routine surroundings. You'll return home glowing.

Devote the day to making your home a warmer, happier place. Take another look at your kitchen, your bath, your cozy bay window. Look at these places not with a critical eye ("Sheesh! That stain needs to go!"), but with a loving one. Ask, "How can I make this corner feel warmer and more fun? How can I add an uplifting touch to that spot?" Here are some suggestions:

- If you love working in the kitchen and enjoy music, too, create a little musical corner in the kitchen. A small cassette player and a collection of your favorite songs is all it takes, but it will keep you humming while you cook.

- If you like to relax on your loveseat or chaise lounge in the bedroom, surround it with comforting objects that please your mind: a basket filled with your favorite books, a bowl of smooth river pebbles for you to run your fingers over, a cuddly stuffed toy, seashells or photographs from a favorite trip.

- If, like me, you like low, dramatic lighting, buy a lovely little lamp and place it in your favorite corner for relaxing. The warm pool of light will soothe your eyes and lure you to relax under its glow.

- Place a bowl of water beside your favorite lounging chair, and float some fresh rose petals and a few drops of rose essential oil in it for a soothing effect.

- Tuck a rolling pin under your bed; just before climbing between the sheets, roll your feet gently along the pin for a mini-massage. Or keep a rolling pin or a foot-roller in your office drawer to use at work.

- If you love to relax in the tub — and who doesn't? — treat yourself to the after-bath luxury of a warm towel. It's easy; all you have to do is install a warming bar in the bathroom.

These little touches — the lamp, the rolling pin, the warming bar — are not expensive or exclusive in themselves. What makes them special is the thoughtfulness you showed yourself in putting them there.

Pamper yourself beautiful. The closest, most intimate space we inhabit is our body. Soothing your skin with the textures and scents it loves is the quickest way to send happy messages surging through your entire being.

- Does your lingerie drawer feel a need for silkier, softer, fresher garments? If so, today's the day! Head for the store, bypass the "discount" sections, and buy yourself some stylish, comfortable lingerie. You'll feel beautiful.

- Is your bathtub surrounded by lotions and potions that will make you feel feminine? If not, why not? Tour a bath-and-body shop, testing out fragrances and creams.

Even if you cannot afford the big bottles, buy a few sachets or trial-sized pots to place around your tub. Make bathing a luxurious experience by giving yourself a bath massage glove, a long-handled brush, aromatic candles, a loofah, salt scrubs, and a special pillow to rest your head on while bathing. None of these are very expensive, yet they can make you feel like a princess.

• If you've been feeling dull lately, buy yourself a new dress, a new scarf, or a new pair of shoes. Or get a new haircut; it symbolizes shedding the old in favor of the new and exciting.

Now you can see that there are dozens of ways to enjoy a day in your own company. But a Me Day is only fun when you spend it without telling yourself you're "stealing" or "grabbing" time. This day, this opportunity to heal and refresh, is yours by right. You deserve every second of that indulgence. And remember: You're doing it so you can make other people happy, too!

Now Extend the Connection

LEARNING TO LOOK AFTER YOURSELF teaches you something magical: the ability to stop expecting others to be artificial, formal, or fake. You are able to give more space to those around you because you understand — firsthand — how good it feels to have that space. And this new, accommodating you evolves into a much happier, much nicer mother, wife, colleague, and friend — all by just being kinder to yourself.

When you're nice, your spouse knows it's okay to sometimes not be in the mood for going out to dinner. Your kids don't always feel obliged to go out for a concert with you when they'd rather spend an evening with their friends. Your friends can feel reassured that you'll understand if they can't call you up more often. Feeling thus liberated from constant obligation, they're all willing to make you happy in return. So keep the generosity coming!

Generous. Hmm.

Wouldn't we all like to be more generous, kinder, nicer — but where's the time? Think again. You'll find that there are dozens of ways to squeeze some goodness into your day, in clever little ways such as these:

In an Instant

YOU CAN BE a more pleasant person just by flashing your widest, brightest smile. Some thoughts on what a smile can do:

- A smile may only last a moment, but its memory can last a lifetime.

- A smile can awaken hope in the bleakest of hearts. You never know how much your smile can mean to a person who doesn't receive one often, so give your smiles away freely, even to strangers.

- When you smile, you're instantly approachable and immediately likeable.

- Best of all, a smile is free; in fact, it is of no use to anyone until it's given away!

- Smile as often as you can, at as many people as you can.

In a Minute or Two

YOU CAN BE A FINER FRIEND. So what if you can never seem to keep your promise to "meet over lunch" or "get together for coffee"? You can be a better friend just while sitting at your desk. Here's how:

- Keep a set of postcards in your bag. Whenever you have two minutes, jot down your thoughts for your friend.

- Return your friend's calls and answer her e-mails immediately. Don't worry that you'll have to spend a long time talking; even if you have only one minute to spare, call her to say you're thinking of her. She'll understand that you have to rush, but she'll also know that you cared enough to pause and say hello.

- Make her day: Send her a bouquet of flowers. All you have to do is pick up the phone, call a florist, and dictate a warm personal message.

- When a friend tells you she's going for a mammogram or sending her child to daycare for the first time, stick a note near your computer to remind yourself to ask how it went — even if only in one sentence on e-mail. She'll be touched that you took the time to ask.

In Five Minutes

YOU CAN BE a nicer neighbor:

- If you're going to the library, ask your neighbor if she has some books you can return or borrow for her.

- If you're baking cookies, bake an extra batch, package it in simple brown paper and raffia, and give it to a neighbor or friend.

- If you're mowing your lawn, mow hers, too. Or if you're clearing the snow from your pavement, shovel it for her, too.

In Ten Minutes

YOU CAN BE a better spouse:

- Give him a foot massage.

- Make tea for the two of you and sip it together — in the pouring rain!

- Sew the missing buttons on his shirt.

- If he's feeling low, give him a hug — or even a loving, thoughtful look — to let him know you understand and are ready to talk about it when he is.

- Pull him close and rest his head on your lap.

- Tell him he looks irresistible. Then...don't resist him.

In Fifteen Minutes

YOU CAN BE a better mom. We all know that the best gift we can give our children is our time. But what if we don't have an hour a day? Don't feel guilty; fifteen minutes can be just as good if you're fully present with your child during that time. Spend the time listening to your child, reading to her, talking to her. Making the most of that time, even for those few precious minutes, can help make her feel mothered and secure in a busy, chaotic world. Here are some fulfilling activities you can share with your children even if you're short of time:

- Cook together. Let your kids handle small jobs, such as mixing and pouring, setting the table, or — if they're a bit older — preparing salad, adding toppings to pizza, or shaping cookies. It's a great way to connect with your family as dinner gets prepared.

- As you prepare dinner, encourage your kids to tell you about their day, their thoughts, their wishes. You could casually ask your child, "What fun stuff have you been wanting to do for a long time now?" If the answer is something doable and reasonably inexpensive, such as a visit to the zoo or a movie, keep that surprise ready for them on the weekend.

• Have a "just-a-minute" session, in which you and your kids get to speak spontaneously on a topic for one full minute. We do this often, and the results are often hilarious. Some topics we've covered are, "If I were a hippopotamus...," " The trouble with clocks...," and "mathematics."

• Similarly, you could pick out a theme and express your thoughts on it together. My son and I like to give each other random topics on a time-limit of ten minutes. We've explored many ideas together: "the world's most beautiful place," "water," "my dream," and many more. We've kept all our writings in a huge file, which we go over together when there's time. It makes for lots of laughter, happy memories, and a wonderful sense of bonding.

• Give your little one an after-bath massage with a good-quality lotion. It's the perfect "mother's touch."

• Don't succumb to the temptation to tell your kids to "go watch TV" so that you're free to cook, clean, pay the bills, or finish your article. Once in a while, postpone the chores and spend a few minutes playing a refreshing board game with them instead.

In One Day

YOU CAN SHOW EVERYONE around you how much you care. Just like you should take a Me Day off, you should also set aside some Us Days to do all the nurturing things you've been meaning to do for the people in your life. Some ideas:

Bond with Your Buddies

- Make time for a just-the-two-of-us evening with your best friend — even if it means giving up something "more important." Stir up some *chai* (see pages 182–84 for recipes), bake cookies, and chat late into the night. Or go to the movies, followed by dinner in the coziest corner of your favorite restaurant.

- Pulled apart by different jobs, different cities? Get creative! Sandy Sheehy, author of *Connecting: The Enduring Power of Female Friendships*, says, "I know women who watch the Oscars together over the phone on opposite coasts."[2]

- Invite your close pals for a sleepover.

- Go on a spa weekend together; you'll not only return glowing, but you'll bring back lovely memories of a healing time spent together.

Take Time for Your Kids

KIDS JUST WANT TO have out-and-out fun. Once in a while, allow them to chalk out an exciting plan of action for the day — within reason, of course. They'll feel like masters of their domain, and everyone will have a blast.

Here are some outdoorsy ideas to choose among:

- Be a kid again in the company of your children. Take them to a theme park, cruise down water slides, swim, and enjoy ice cream, cotton candy, and popcorn together.

- Go out to the zoo, or visit the circus, carnival, or magic show that might be running in your town. Then go to lunch, followed by whatever else your kids want to do.

- Pull out a local map and drive to some place you haven't explored yet.

- Be bold! Take a day off from work and spend it with your kids. The advantage: You can take them to a museum or a planetarium without having to brave traffic snarl-ups and long lines. You could also take them to an interesting, knowledge-enhancing facility such as a bread factory or a coin mint.

- Erect a tent made from old bedsheets in your backyard and have a picnic there.

- Skip rope, fly kites, play hide-and-go-seek, and, of course, have a lavish spread of treats.

Not in the mood for going out? There's still plenty you can do: Stay indoors and share some intimate moments; settle down in the family room and talk about your memories, hopes, and dreams. For ideas on what to talk about, pick up a copy of *The Mom and Dad Conversation Piece* (Ballantine Books, 1997) or *Who We Are* (New World Library, 2000) by Bret Nicholaus and Paul Lowrie. These delicious books feature hundreds of interesting, heartwarming questions such as these: "What's the most memorable road you've ever driven on? What was your favorite grade in school? If you could add one room to the house that would serve any unique purpose you desired, what would the room be?"[3] Or, even more fun, make up your own questions and jot down the memorable answers in a family journal.

Spend the Day with Your Spouse

- Make this day sheer fun. Enjoy something childlike together. Make paper boats, watch a circus, or play Monopoly. You're never more "together" than when you're both having pure, un"adult"erated fun.

- Think up and complete a home project together. The keyword here is not "project" or "complete"; it's "together."

- Ditch the project! Halfway to Home Depot, take a U-turn and head for the video store. Bring home *When Harry Met Sally* and enjoy it together. (More must-watch romantic films: *The Bridges of Madison County, Gone with the Wind, Ghost, Falling in Love, Love Story, Casablanca, Out of Africa, A Walk in the Clouds, An Affair to Remember, Wuthering Heights.*) Or do a movie marathon: one movie of your choice followed by one of his.

- So what if it isn't his birthday or your anniversary? Give each other gifts "just because." You give him a collection of poems, and let him think of a creative gift for you. Don't worry too much about cost and choice; think from the heart. The beauty of romance is in the spontaneity of its gestures.

- Speaking of gifts, the art of presenting a gift is special, too. Have a treasure hunt. Scatter gifts all over your home, and give him clues that lead to the treasures. Feeling naughty? Let one of the clues be "kiss and tell." He gives you a kiss, and you tell him where the next clue is. (In fact, try a fun, "clean-themed" treasure-hunt with your kids as well — they'll be thrilled!)

- Reserve a corner table at the most romantic restaurant in town. Over hot pasta and cool wine, talk to each other late into the night — just like the first time.

- Allow yourselves to sit — simply sit — in companionable silence for a while. Under the stars, by the seashore, in a chapel — find a quiet spot and, holding hands, take in the beautiful silence that calls out to you.

• Spend time in the garden. Plant a tree together, then nurture it and watch it grow, just like your love.

Long-Term Deposits in the Relationship Bank

WITH EACH GIFT OF GOODNESS you give to others, you'll add golden coins of gratitude to your emotional bank. Can there be a better way to "get rich" quick?

The Best Gifts to Give Your Friends

• a sympathetic ear

• positive advice

• the knowledge that you're always there for them

• the reassurance that, despite your commitments to work and family, their place in your heart is special and unique

During times when you find friendship slipping way down the ladder of your priorities, remind yourself of the friendship thoughts that great men and women have given us:

> *The best mirror is an old friend.*
>
> — George Herbert

> *A friend may well be reckoned the masterpiece of Nature.*
>
> — Ralph Waldo Emerson

> *My friends are my estate.*
>
> — Emily Dickinson

*My Friend is that one whom I can associate with my
choicest thought.*

— Henry David Thoreau

Of all possessions a friend is the most precious.

— Herodotus

*Each friend represents a world in us, a world possibly not
born until they arrive, and it is only by this meeting that a
new world is born.*

— Anaïs Nin

Most importantly, remember that a lull in your relationship
doesn't mean you've lost a friend. You can always reconnect and
pick up the threads where you left off; that's the unique beauty of
friendship.

How to Cherish Your Children

"I DO NOT LOVE him because he is good," said Nobel laureate
Rabindranath Tagore, "but because he is my little child."[4] What
a powerful way of saying why we love our children!

While we all interpret and understand parenting differently,
I've found that some tried-and-tested advice can help anyone be a
more nurturing mother. My favorite tips:

- Never, never, ever be sarcastic to your children. Words
  can leave scars for life.

- Take the time to talk with your kids about things that
  matter to them. Simple questions and comments — such
  as "How was the basketball game?" "Did you enjoy your
  school lunch?" or "I like your new shirt!" — will make
  your kids feel you care, giving them a sense of security.

- Make your children feel as if their ideas and opinions count for something. Saying "What do kids know?" is a put-down, and children are very sensitive to such ridicule.

- Cultivate the art of listening without being judgmental. Make your kids feel they can confide in you — and be sure you keep their confidences!

- If your kids do something wrong, don't just yell at them and punish them. Take the time to explain to them patiently what they did wrong and why they shouldn't have done it. Once they truly understand your reasons, they'll be more willing to behave well.

- Honor the promises you make to your children.

Being a Wholesome Wife

HERE'S HOW I LOOK AT MARRIAGE: Watch a gymnast walking on a balance beam — how she sometimes leans left and sometimes right, just so she can stay on the beam. Now imagine that the gymnast has to lock arms with another person, and then tread the beam. To me, this is being married: treading a balancing beam that sits atop a steep, rocky cliff. You'll stumble, and you'll lurch — but as long as you hold on to each other's hands, the journey will be worthwhile.

Some Simple Rules of Balance

When You Stumble

HAVE YOU SEEN a couple that never fights? Neither have I. But it's one thing to fight and make up, and quite another to let the hostile feelings fester. The next time you exchange words, play by the rules:

Do:

- Express your anger constructively; bottling it up can sometimes be as destructive as letting it out.

- Think solutions — not accusations. Helen Backer, a seventy-three-year-old retired advertising professional from Missouri, has been married for more than thirty years. She says, "Speak up at home when you need help with the load. When I was first married, it was difficult for my husband to accept the fact that he had to be responsible for some of the household tasks, but I hung in there and insisted."

- Remember that, no matter how strongly you disagree, you love him and he loves you.

Don't:

- Call him names — however tempted you might be.

- Hurl the past at him as a weapon.

- Walk away in a huff or turn over and sleep, leaving an issue unresolved.

Let your argument become a tool for resolution, not a weapon for deeper conflict.

In Steady Times

Do:

- Look good for him — without losing your identity. You don't have to have silicone implants to make him happy; just a clean, sweet-smelling you is enough to drive him crazy with desire. Besides, you'll inspire him to look good for you, too.

- Savor little pleasures together: Cuddle up in front of the television to watch a film, share breakfast in bed on a weekend, give each other a massage.

- Give each other some breathing space. Remember the immortal words of Kahlil Gibran in *The Prophet:* "Let there be spaces in your togetherness...."[5]

- Create adventure in the mundane. Vary your routine even if you cannot afford to take expensive vacations. Try something new regularly: a new restaurant, a new distribution of chores, a new way to make love.

- Be hopelessly romantic. Say "Tumi ho ichema," "Ich liebe dich" — "I love you" — in as many languages as you can, as many times as you can. Pick out a favorite photograph of you and him together, then have it laminated into a bookmark. Write him syrupy love letters — even if you've been married twenty-four years. Spray your note with natural perfume, and tuck it in a place where he'll find it first thing in the morning. You're guaranteed at least a hug...if not more!

Don't:

- Don't try to change each other. Instead, when you feel frustrated with some of his traits, try to think of all the good and positive things about him; you'll find plenty.

- The old advice "Don't go to bed angry" sounds clichéd, but it's essential. Bottled up resentment can cause an ugly, hurtful explosion — so don't keep it inside! Sometimes it's a great idea to let go of your ego and follow Ogden Nash's advice on how to resolve a conflict:

    To keep love brimming in the loving cup, When you're wrong admit it and when you're right shut up![6]

IN THESE SMALL, simple ways, you can breathe fresh energy into all your relationships. And when the returns start to come — in the form of smiles, hugs, letters, gifts, and abundant gestures of love — you'll realize that the time you took "off" for yourself and the people in your life was worth its weight in gold.

Let me close with a thread of thought that runs common to all the relationships in the world: Relationships are about emotions, and emotions are not math. This is one arena of life where you can — and should — occasionally forget logic and be recklessly good, randomly kind, and impulsively affectionate.

And, oh! Before you rush off to plant a wet kiss on a surprised cheek, don't forget to disconnect that cell phone.

Chapter Summary and Resources

- Take a break from technology and rediscover the joy of personal communication. For inspiration, give yourself an evening with Gary Chapman's can't-put-it-down book, *The Five Love Languages: How to Express Heartfelt Commitment to Your Mate* (Northfield Publishing, 1992).

- In order to be able to love others, first love yourself.

- Don't wait until you have the time and money to give yourself a healing vacation; take time out to enjoy the simple things.

- Once a week, once a month, or as often as your schedule permits, enjoy a Me Day, taking time out for yourself.

- When you begin to feel centered within yourself, reach out to others.

- Little acts of kindness and simple gestures of love can make those around you feel cherished. Besides doing small favors for those around you, think about giving to people you have never met. The Better Business Bureau's Wise Giving Alliance Website (www.give.org) has useful tips on how to help those in need.

- Don't sacrifice your personal relationships on the altar of other commitments. Take a day out with friends and family; you'll be glad you did. Or give in to impulse and take a last-minute weekend trip. Check out Websites such as hotwire.com and lastminutedeals.com for travel bargains. Browse magazines such as *Spa Magazine*

THOUGHTS FROM CARLA SIDES,
HOMEMAKER, 42

Here are the most important things I've learned about relationships with the people in my life:

Friends:

The people you surround yourself with will shape who you become in the next five years.

Your friends will be the peer group that influences your values and your purchases.

Spouse:

The best marriages I have observed are those based on friendship and intellectual equality.

Grandparents:

The experiences they share and what they teach you about a life well lived are more valuable than you may imagine.

Children:

Respect is a two-way street. The more you give it to your children, the more they will give it to you.

or *Healing Retreats & Spas* for ideas on how to recharge and renew.

- In all your close relationships, respect the relationship, treasure it, and learn to give people their space.

THOUGHTS FROM NANCY BERTLE, HOMEMAKER, 45

I think the secret of a successful relationship with your spouse or partner is this: Stick with each other through the tough times. My husband and I have forged a deeper emotional bond while wading through difficulties. When you do that, you're less likely to say, "He doesn't help around the house," or "I'm bored with him." Your love for each other overcomes those things.

Another essential in the recipe for a great relationship: Keep the romance alive! My husband has a way with giving gifts. He doesn't buy me diamonds or expensive clothing. But he likes to think up simple surprises for me, in ways that say "I care." On my birthday last year, he gave me a sachet of aroma candles and essential oils. In the evening, he lit the candles and gave me a back rub and a foot massage with those wonderful oils. It was tremendously touching — in the true sense of the word.

CHAPTER 6

Repose

How to Relax and Revive Your Body and Mind

*You must learn to be still in the midst of activity
and to be vibrantly alive in repose.*

— INDIRA GANDHI

Drip, drip, drip. The soft but constant sound permeates my consciousness as I slice bell peppers for dinner. With each passing minute, the "drip" amplifies itself many decibels, until finally it explodes in my head. Before I can help it, I'm yelling, "Stop, stop, STOP! I can't take it any more!" I sink down on the couch, holding my head in my hands. Later I'm ashamed of my outburst, and at a loss for an answer when my son asks, "Just because a tap was leaking, Ma?"

If you've experienced a similar situation at some point, I'm sure you know that such flare-ups don't happen "just because." They are almost always a combined explosion of several small but long-pent-up stresses.

Stress Plus Stress Plus Stress...

THOUGH STRESS MANIFESTS itself in many complex ways, it nearly always starts with simple things: the niggling little discomforts and disorderly acts of daily life. Having to rush through the shower, missing out on breakfast, forgetting to call a friend back, being late for an appointment — slowly, the combined weight of these "not-dones" and "half-dones" begins to bog down the body, mind, and heart. The resulting bodily miseries, mental blocks, and mood swings spell s-t-r-e-s-s.

Each time I analyze stress this way, I start feeling really good. The reason is simple: I tell myself that, after all, if stress is made up of such small elements, there must be simple ways in which to tackle it.

Here are some practical, no-fail stress-busting strategies I've devised over the years:

Don't Do What You Don't Have to Do

WHAT HAPPENS when you put too much on your plate and feel obligated to eat it all? You get indigestion. It's the same with stress: Make too many commitments, struggle to keep them all, and — oops! You've sentenced yourself to a lifetime of tension.

Yet we seem addicted to our commitments. A young marketing executive once told me, "The most difficult part of my week is Sunday mornings; there's nothing to do, and that makes me extremely restless." No wonder, then, that studies on stress are constantly coming up with depressing data. Here are some scary findings:

- Three-quarters of all visits to the doctor are for stress-related illnesses.

- People who experience high levels of anxiety are four to five times more likely to die of a heart attack or stroke.

- Stress-related ailments such as chronic pain, headaches, and high blood pressure are thought to be responsible for half of all absences from work.

- The cost of job stress in North America is estimated in the billions annually; this includes related costs of absenteeism, lost productivity, and insurance claims.

- Many surveys have confirmed that three-quarters of all workers say they feel stressed during a typical workday.

POSITIVE THOUGHTS FOR POSITIVE DAYS

Let every dawn of morning be to you as the beginning of life, and every setting sun be to you as its close: then let every one of these short lives leave its sure record of some kindly thing done for others — some goodly strength or knowledge gained for yourselves.

— J. Ruskin

Hope is itself a species of happiness, and, perhaps, the chief happiness which this world affords.   — Samuel Johnson

May dawn, as the proverb goes, bring happy tidings coming from her mother night.   — Aeschylus

Write it in your heart that every day is the best day of the year.

— Ralph Waldo Emerson

I am one who eats breakfast gazing at morning glories.

— Matsuo Basho

Every day in every way, I am getting better and better.

— Emile Coué

The time to relax is when you don't have time for it.

— Sidney J. Harris

With such restorative thoughts to launch you into a glorious new day, who could stop you from being the joyful, restful person you want to be?

Halt! Just for a moment, think about the ways in which you over-commit yourself to people and things. On a piece of paper, draw a circle and divide it into two portions: one depicting the percentage of your day you spend doing things you want to do, and the other demarcating the percentage you spend doing things you have to do. Which of these chunks is larger?

If you find an appallingly high ratio of "I-have-tos" in your life, don't despair. Here are three ways to start reducing the pile on your plate right away:

1. Say the "N" word. Picture this: You've been working so hard that you've almost forgotten what the word "vacation" means. Finally, you decide to book tickets for a refreshing weekend in Aspen. Then the phone rings. It's a prospective client, with "an offer you can't resist." A familiar rush of adrenaline begins to course through your veins. You find yourself saying, "Of course I'll do it." Later, you wonder what you gained and what you lost by saying "yes" to that project. But by then, you're already committed.

Here's an easy way to deal with the situation: Next time a persuasive client, boss, or friend asks you to take on "just one more" task, don't rush to say "yes." Ask for time to think — even if only for a few minutes. Then pause to ask yourself this question: "How will agreeing to this request affect the quality of rest, nourishment, and relationships in my life?" If the answer makes you unhappy, brace yourself to say a polite but firm "no."

2. Pause before you pay. I know, I know. That snazzy little laptop is to die for. It has a huge amount of memory and a multi-function drive to play movies or write CDs. What's more, you're getting a good deal. The only thing is: You know you're going to use the laptop barely ten minutes a day, just to check your e-mail, and you already have a decent personal computer and a DVD player. So you don't really need that laptop, you desire it —

temporarily ignoring the fact that this new toy will cost you money, take up space, and require maintenance. In other words, it will require you to commit precious resources that you could use on other, truly essential items.

Beware: Temptation loves to come your way in irresistible disguises! It will beckon you in the form of an alluring dress, an attractive credit-card offer, a sexy new car. Be dispassionate. Take time to work out a commitment-versus-comfort ratio, and you'll be able to make wiser decisions.

3. **Stop before you speak.** A woman I hadn't even invited to my home (she came with a friend I had called over for a party) remarked, "I just love the music of Pink Floyd." And before I could stop myself, I said, "Oh, me too. In fact I have the entire Pink Floyd collection, including some rare numbers." You can guess what happened next: She asked to see my collection,

GIVE YOUR BODY A STRESS TEST

The sages of ancient India said: "A well-used body is a relaxed body. Learn the art of using your body well: Don't overuse, underuse, misuse, or abuse it." If your bodily aches and pains are making you irritable and unhappy, ask yourself some quick questions. Are you:

- Exercising too much, standing most of the day, or staying up late? (That's overuse.)

- Spending most of your day sitting in a chair? (That's underuse.)

- Slouching or reading in dim light? (That's misuse.)

- Delaying or missing meals, snacking on junk food, or smoking and drinking? (That's abuse.)

Once you've identified the origins of your physical discomfort, you'll find it easier to do something about it.

borrowed some of the rare tapes, and never retu

too caught up in my hyper-busy life to chase he

and then she moved to another continent. I need

tapes, had I not spoken without thinking.

This is just one of the ways in which words

about it, and you'll realize that tactless or impuls

always come back to haunt you. So, just for too

intervals of silence. Speak only when necessary;

a lot of hassle just by keeping quiet.

With all these extra commitments, items,

an exit from your life, you're guaranteed to star

addition, you'll be able to free up time, ener

things that truly deserve your attention. Which

next vital step in freeing yourself of stress:

Don't Postpone What You Have to

IN OTHER WORDS, don't procrastinate. The

the *Cambridge Advanced Learner's Dictionary* defines

tinate" as "to keep delaying something that

because it is unpleasant or boring."[1]

The key words in this definition, I think,

Let's face it: There are things in life that you

doing. Dishes have to be washed, household it

in working condition, library books have to be

do them and get them over with? Take the inc

faucet, for instance. Had I taken the trouble to

it two weeks ago, the problem would hav

forgotten within two minutes. But because I all I

it spun out of proportion.

I invite you to make time for your "have-to-d

out, however tiny they seem. Put them in words.

waiting for your attention at this moment. Here

temporarily ignoring the fact that this new toy will cost you money, take up space, and require maintenance. In other words, it will require you to commit precious resources that you could use on other, truly essential items.

Beware: Temptation loves to come your way in irresistible disguises! It will beckon you in the form of an alluring dress, an attractive credit-card offer, a sexy new car. Be dispassionate. Take time to work out a commitment-versus-comfort ratio, and you'll be able to make wiser decisions.

3. **Stop before you speak.** A woman I hadn't even invited to my home (she came with a friend I had called over for a party) remarked, "I just love the music of Pink Floyd." And before I could stop myself, I said, "Oh, me too. In fact I have the entire Pink Floyd collection, including some rare numbers." You can guess what happened next: She asked to see my collection,

GIVE YOUR BODY A STRESS TEST

The sages of ancient India said: "A well-used body is a relaxed body. Learn the art of using your body well: Don't overuse, underuse, misuse, or abuse it." If your bodily aches and pains are making you irritable and unhappy, ask yourself some quick questions. Are you:

- Exercising too much, standing most of the day, or staying up late? (That's overuse.)

- Spending most of your day sitting in a chair? (That's underuse.)

- Slouching or reading in dim light? (That's misuse.)

- Delaying or missing meals, snacking on junk food, or smoking and drinking? (That's abuse.)

Once you've identified the origins of your physical discomfort, you'll find it easier to do something about it.

borrowed some of the rare tapes, and never returned them. I was too caught up in my hyper-busy life to chase her beyond a point, and then she moved to another continent. I needn't have lost those tapes, had I not spoken without thinking.

This is just one of the ways in which words cause stress. Think about it, and you'll realize that tactless or impulsive remarks almost always come back to haunt you. So, just for today, practice small intervals of silence. Speak only when necessary; you'll save yourself a lot of hassle just by keeping quiet.

With all these extra commitments, items, and words making an exit from your life, you're guaranteed to start feeling calmer. In addition, you'll be able to free up time, energy, and money for things that truly deserve your attention. Which brings me to the next vital step in freeing yourself of stress:

Don't Postpone What You Have to Do

IN OTHER WORDS, don't procrastinate. The Internet edition of the *Cambridge Advanced Learner's Dictionary* defines the word "procrastinate" as "to keep delaying something that must be done, often because it is unpleasant or boring."[1]

The key words in this definition, I think, are "must be done." Let's face it: There are things in life that you and I cannot avoid doing. Dishes have to be washed, household items have to be kept in working condition, library books have to be returned. Why not do them and get them over with? Take the incident of the leaking faucet, for instance. Had I taken the trouble to buy a washer and fix it two weeks ago, the problem would have been solved and forgotten within two minutes. But because I allowed it to build up, it spun out of proportion.

I invite you to make time for your "have-to-dos" today. Spell them out, however tiny they seem. Put them in words. Count how many are waiting for your attention at this moment. Here is a sample list:

- The laundry pile is approaching the height of Mount Rainier.

- Three library books have now been overdue for a week.

- You really do need to pull out those dandelions before they set seed.

- You need some containers for the kitchen. Several items are lying around in plastic packets, tied up with rubber bands; they look ugly, and they often spill when opened.

- At least ten week-old e-mails are sitting in your "In" box. If you don't reply soon enough, you could upset a friend or lose a contract.

What has this analysis done for you? On the minus side, it tells you that your life is littered with little time bombs of discomfort, each waiting to explode. But on the plus side, you now know what those time bombs are, so you can systematically defuse each of them.

So tomorrow, when you're going to the supermarket, remember to haul the library books along. While waiting for the eggs to boil, you can run downstairs and pop a load of clothes into the washer. Ah, just thinking about it makes you feel much better, doesn't it?

Make lists; they help you remember and focus on the tasks that await your attention. Identify five little things-to-do today — or in the near future. Then plan on doing them.

Don't go at it hammer and tongs, though. You don't have to pull the last of those billion dandelions today. And you don't have to suffer sore fingers from typing ten essay-type e-mails tonight. Start with five dandelions, two e-mails, one laundry load. Do a few more tomorrow, and some the day after. Go slowly, but steadily.

Squeeze these small chores in between other, more "important" ones. Learning to manage your time this way is an art, and it takes time to learn. Just don't give up.

Don't Race Against Time, Fall in Step with It

TO HELP YOU START managing your time better, here are some tips. Follow them, and they'll take your life from chaotic to calm in the course of a chockablock day.

In the Morning

- If you can summon the willpower, wake up early. Not only does this give you extra time to get organized, but it's tremendously healing, too. All of nature is waking up: birds, flowers, sunshine. The crisp morning air, alive with fresh energy, prompted Benjamin Franklin to say, "The early morning hath gold in its mouth." The healers of India agree. They call this period *amrita bela,* Sanskrit for "a time filled with nectar." Wake up early, and you'll reap rich rewards all day long.

- Don't spring out of bed as soon as you open your eyes. This might seem like a waste of time, but it isn't. If you take just a minute or two to create a space in your mind for the day ahead, you'll notice a change in your attitude throughout the day. Think sunny thoughts. Take a deep breath, inviting fresh energy and vitality into your being. Slowly exhale, breathing out stale stress.

- Before you leave the bedroom, take a minute to make your bed. You'll be pleased to come back to it in the evening.

- In the shower, run a quick mental scan of the day ahead. Are you going to be ultra-busy? If so, number your tasks for the day from one to five in order of importance. Plan on completing the most urgent and important ones first, then move lower down the list. Do you see chores that can easily be postponed to a few days later? If so, cross them out in your head. You'll feel instantly relieved.

In the Evening

- While driving home from work, check your car for gas. If you're low, fill up now so that you won't waste valuable minutes in the morning.

- Monday through Thursday night, take five minutes before bedtime to select your clothes and shoes for the next morning. Iron the clothes and lay them out. Polish your shoes. If weather is an important variable in the region where you live, it's a good idea to glance at the evening news and plan your outerwear accordingly.

- While preparing dinner, run through the breakfast menu in your mind, then check the fridge and pantry for ingredients you will need. To save time, pour out cereal in bowls, slice and refrigerate or freeze fruit, and lay out protein bars, cups, and dishes on the breakfast table, restaurant style. These small steps will make sure you don't have to scramble in the morning.

- You can also plan on a hot lunch for the next day by setting up stew in a slow-cooker overnight.

- Go to bed early. A good night's rest will help you wake up fresh, and you'll be able to go about your day's business more efficiently and cheerfully. If you tend to go to bed late, gradually move your bedtime closer to 10:00 P.M. at the rate of fifteen minutes each night. Shift gears into calming activities as bedtime draws near: Avoid violent or excessively stimulating entertainment. Instead, listen to soothing music or take a relaxing warm bath to lull your senses.

On the Weekend

- Ah! The weekend is your chance to do some real planning and organizing. Give it some time now, and you'll reap the rewards for a long time to come.

- Make a list of things you can buy in bulk: toothpaste, detergent, greeting cards, stamps, wrapping paper. Then go shopping for them. This saves a tremendous amount of time, energy, and trouble.

- Find a central spot in your home and call it "Paper Place." Put a large basket there, and make it a receptacle for all your mail, e-mail or Internet printouts, and bills. Sort and clear these out when you have time.

- It's easy to forget small repairs and things you need to buy. Put reminders on your fridge: "sew missing button on blue shirt," "stitch up hem of pink skirt," "replace the attic bulb."

- If you want to enjoy your weekends to the fullest, plan to finish all your housecleaning and grocery-shopping chores by Thursday, setting aside an evening for each job if you work away from home. Then enjoy a Free Friday!

At the Workplace

- Back up all your computer files — at home and at work. Here's a scary statistic from hotmail.com: one in every five computers is infected with a virus. Why wait for yours to be struck? Copy your files now!

- Organize your e-mail. Use the Address Book folders to list e-mails by groups — To Do, To Reply, To Call, for example. You can also organize people by groups in your mailbox: family, friends, colleagues, and so on. This is also an important tip to implement on your home computer.

- When it comes to paperwork, use the "divide and conquer" approach! Don't let loose papers float around on your desk — it's amazing how many of them pile up if unchecked, and how quickly. Tuck them, as you go along, into clearly labeled folders. Or, set aside a few minutes first or last thing in your day to do this — your desk will look clean and attractive, and you'll feel supremely organized. This is another good tip to keep in mind for your home office.

- Few things in life are as frustrating as that frantic last-minute search for a stray piece of paper on which you jotted down an important phone number or address. Keep your planner handy, and record every small bit of information into it for easy access.

- Think beyond comb, brush, and lipstick. Don't forget to carry some stamps, a few envelopes, a pen, and some loose change in your purse. You'll be glad you did — especially when you feel like writing a letter or paying bills during your lunch hour or while grabbing a cup of tea or coffee on your break.

• When you walk into your workplace knowing it's going to be one of those crazily busy days, try this strategy — focus on one task at a time. For each job well done, give yourself a small reward. If you don't have time to take even a small breather during your day, make it up to yourself in the evening — catch a movie, dine out, or spend a luxurious hour in the bath.

Comfort Yourself with Good Buys

BUT, HEY, STRESS RELIEF shouldn't be solely about juggling time and completing chores. How about helping yourself to some comfort, too? One way to increase your comfort level is to make sure you have the things you need before you need them.

Here's an example of what I mean: You're at home and the phone rings. It is your boss calling: An unexpected client meeting has been scheduled in twenty minutes. Panicky, you rummage through your closet and pull out a pair of trousers. Shucks! The zipper won't close. You hurriedly iron a dress, trying not to remember that you've worn the same dress for the past three meetings. You manage to scramble out the door in time, only to realize that it's raining. You pop back in to grab an umbrella, then you realize that you trashed the old broken one and never found time to buy a new one. Muttering in frustration, you step out in the pouring rain, already five minutes late.

The moral of the story: Sometimes it pays to be a go-getter. Go get yourself those items, big and small, that you need — really need — for smooth everyday living. This practical step will make your life incredibly easier, lifting tons of stress from your body and mind.

Here are a few of the everyday things that spell "comfort" for me:

- At least two good dresses, washed and ironed — ready to go out when I am, even on five minutes' notice.

- A comfortable, back-friendly, adjustable office chair.

- Smooth pens, sharpened pencils, clips, notepads, stapler, letter-opener and other stationary essentials in my office desk drawer.

- A pantry filled at all times with basic supplies, such as good-quality olive oil, pasta, herbs, spices, pickles, cookies, and honey.

- A set of good knives and a pair of sharp scissors in the kitchen.

- A message pad and a pen next to each telephone in the house.

DON'T SAY "WHAT IF"

"What if I don't get the job?"

"What if this roller coaster crashes?"

"What if I miss the bus?"

A lot of our stress exists solely in our imagination. Those feelings of dread and anxiety are terribly toxic. Worse, they have the potential to become real. British playwright George Bernard Shaw said, "In this world, danger is always present for those who are afraid of it."

Stop worrying and do something concrete about your worries. Walk your dog. Take out the trash. Shovel snow. Clean out a cupboard. Knead dough — pummel it into a fantastic base for pizza. Play frisbee — and imagine that you're physically flinging your worries away each time you throw. Dump your stress in the compost bin: A vigorous thirty minutes of gardening will give your body a healthy workout, and your mind a much-needed break.

- Comfortable cotton and flannel pajamas for the night.

- Clean bed linen, extra pillows, and spare toothbrushes for unexpected guests.

- A reliable flashlight and a stock of matches, candles, lanterns, food, and water in case the lights go out on a stormy day.

- Good garden tools. After struggling to prepare a flower bed with a blunt old shovel, I finally went out and bought a stainless-steel claw that fit perfectly in my hand. Within an hour, I had lovely lobelias and pretty petunias singing in my garden.

See what I mean? These are things that say "reach out, and I'm right here." They give you the joy of easy living. How reassuring! How comforting!

So make a master list of all the things that will make your life smoother. Then one by one, based on your available budget and time, make your purchases. Don't worry if you can't immediately afford everything. The great thing is that you now know what you really need, and this awareness will help you save up for those things. Also, you'll be able to resist the temptation to buy things you can do without.

When Stress Strikes

SLICING HUGE CHUNKS of stress out of your life can actually be quite easy. But let's face it: Sometimes no amount of planning and organizing can keep stress away. "Down days" are part of life, and there are times when we feel truly blue. What to do when that happens? Plenty! Here are some soft-and-sunny suggestions to help you sail away from stress.

Drink Water

NEXT TIME YOU FEEL TIRED, drink a tall glass of water. I know of no simpler way to feel better in an instant. Those eight fluid ounces of water seep into your system to:

- Replenish moisture in your body,

- Flush away accumulated debris and waste from your cells,

- Assist your digestive process,

- Rejuvenate your organs and help them function better,

- Put the glow back in your skin, and

- Help you resist the urge to eat; we often mistake thirst for hunger.

Binge on Healthy, Satisfying Snacks

WHEN WE'RE STRESSED, we like to eat. Let me amend that: We have to eat. But over time, I've discovered some delicious alternatives to chips and doughnuts. Here's my list of foods that comfort body and mind without adding up empty calories:

Fresh fruits and vegetables: carrots, corn, beans, greens, bananas, apples, peaches, grapes, oranges, melons, and berries. Add spice and flavor to your bountiful platter of fresh produce by sprinkling it with a spice called *Chaat Masala* (snack spice). You'll find it in stores that sell foodstuff from India. Made from powdered raw mango, black pepper, rock salt, and coriander seeds, this spice is absolutely delicious rubbed on grilled corn-on-the-cob, too.

Nuts: almonds, cashews, pecans, peanuts — all raw or roasted but unsalted, and preferably whole. These are all good sources of protein, which boosts energy and gives a feeling of satisfaction even if you don't eat a big amount. For added taste and energy, you can stir a few of these nuts into a small bottle of honey (all except peanuts, which don't taste great with honey).

Pappadums: The Indian store again! Pappadums are crunchy snacks served before a meal in India. Made from lentils and spices, they can be quite addictive. You can buy a packet of raw pappadums in many flavors, then either deep-fry or roast them. I recommend roasting, for better flavor and less fat. It takes less than five minutes to roast a few pappadums on your stove: Hold them with a pair of tongs and roast them directly over the flame, turning them quickly; they take only a few seconds to fluff up and become crunchy. If you have an electric range, you'll need to be slightly quicker in turning them over, since resting the pappadums directly on the coil can cause them to become charred within seconds. Though delicious on their own, these roasted pappadums can be pepped up with a generous topping of sprouted mung beans, finely chopped tomatoes, onions, and cucumbers on them.

Whole-grain bread: Rub it with juicy garlic, then dip it in warm olive oil that has been seasoned with freshly ground black pepper. Don't limit yourself to plain olive oil, though; you'll find a bounty of herb-infused oils in good stores, so try out different varieties.

A glass of refreshing iced tea with a bowl of fresh sliced fruit: In the summer months, a cooling watermelon slush is a special treat. Just slice watermelon, add a few ice cubes, and blend in a mixer. Stir in some cinnamon and dust sugar on it if you like.

Five whole-grain crackers, each topped with a smidgen of cream cheese: Fresh celery with cream cheese or carrots dipped in sour cream with dill weed is a healthful and delicious treat.

A small box of raisins. A great source of natural energy, raisins contain disease-preventing plant chemicals and contribute toward fulfilling your daily quota of fruit consumption.

Send Stress Packing with a Touch of Love

WHEN YOU ARE TIRED after a long day and you need some tender loving care, your body craves warmth and touch. So what if you can't afford a spa massage? Here are some terrific do-it-yourself ways to heal your body:

- Moisten a flat cotton pad with warm water and place it below your eyes; it's wonderfully soothing. Cool slices of cucumber over the eyes are greatly comforting, too.

- After you make tea, soak the used tea bags in chilled water for a few minutes, then place them over your

WHEN YOU PLAY, STRESS RUNS AWAY

Once in a while, be a child again:

- Jump on a mini-trampoline! It is energizing and uplifting, and it makes you happy like a child. Or, if you're lucky enough to have one around, try a full-sized trampoline. Do all the tricks you did as a kid. Ask a friend to jump with you and fall together. Jump opposite each other and see how high you can go. You'll fall in a pile of giggles. My friend Katie Farnam Conolly says, "Recently, we were visiting with friends who had children — and a trampoline. After all the kids went to bed, we adults got on the trampoline; I became a child again! So did our friends. It was a blast!"

- Get wet! In India, we have a festival called Holi, which is celebrated in a riot of color. Men and women, rich and poor, old and young — everyone is out on the streets throwing handfuls of red, blue, yellow, green, and pink powder on each other, dropping water balloons from terraces, and chasing each other with Super-Soakers. The air is vibrant with energy and laughter. It's a time for letting your hair down, forgetting your grudges, and shedding your shyness. Bring out the child in you: Play super-soaker with your kids today!

• Tie both ends of a good-quality bed sheet to two sturdy tree branches. Once you've tested its security to hold your weight, snuggle up in your hammock with a delicious book. Or curl up with a good magazine, such as *Organic Style*, *Natural Home*, or *Real Simple*. Each issue of these magazines is filled with ideas that will inspire you to live healthfully, naturally, and happily. You'll feel like a child again sitting in your homemade hammock-fort.

• Do a spot of fun gardening with your kids. If you don't have your own, enlist your neighbors' energetic child for an hour or so! Together, prepare a soil-bed or container with soil-mix and water, then get your hands dirty digging holes, looking for worms, pulling weeds, sowing seeds and planting saplings. Reveling thus in the joy of nature, childlike, will nip your stresses in the bud!.

• Do a rumba. Or invent a dance of your own — and call it "Funba."

tired eyelids for an immensely relaxing experience. The tannin in the tea does the trick. You can also use the tea bags warm, allowing them to cool down to a comfortable temperature before placing them on your eyes.

• Rest a hot water bottle on your belly, chest, or back— ah, so comforting!

• Soak a large fluffy towel in warm water. Then wring it out well and wipe your face and arms gently with it. For an even more exquisite sensation, infuse the towel with your favorite essential oil. I love lavender and rose, but you could try chamomile, bergamot, or peppermint.

- Rub warm, herb-infused oil into your scalp. Then wrap a warm, damp towel around your head for thirty minutes. Take a shower afterward.

- Fill a footbath with warm water, and add two to three drops of mint essential oil. Soak your feet in this bath, and feel the tension drain away.

- Pour two teaspoons of olive oil into a small bowl and add two drops of rose, neroli, or peppermint essential oil. Massage the soles of your feet with this aromatic blend for a supremely calming experience.

Try Vitamin S

"S" IS FOR SMILE. A popular Canadian television show for children called *Today's Special* defines a smile as "just a frown upside down." The simple act of relaxing your face into a smile is an affirmation of hope, a message to yourself saying, "Things happen, and I'm ready to sail through them." Try it the next time you're in a traffic jam or a tough meeting. Take a long, deep breath and smile. Let the smile begin with your lips and spread across your entire face, your whole body, your very being. It takes seconds to practice, it's free, and it makes you feel immediately, infinitely relaxed. Besides, it takes only seventeen muscles to smile, but forty-three to frown — so smiling is far easier to do!

Get Close to Someone

WALK UP TO SOMEONE YOU LOVE, put your arms around them, and ask them to do the same to you. This is called a hug, and it is the warmest, most comforting feeling in the world.

If something is bothering you, phone a friend and have a heart-to-heart. Between picking up the receiver and putting it down, your problem will shrink many sizes. The saying "multiply your joys and divide your sorrows" is the basis of friendship. After unburdening your heart to a friend, you'll feel lighthearted and bright.

Feeling friendless and alone? No problem. Find comfort in a crowd. Popcorn at the movies, plays, concerts, magic shows — with so many irresistible options, you really needn't feel alone. Click on www.citysearch.com for a listing of local events, and get yourself a ticket to smile.

Get Some Comic Relief

THEY DON'T CALL LAUGHTER "the best medicine" for nothing. Feelings of mirth and moroseness cannot coexist; when you're laughing out loud, you simply can't be sad.

Yes, it isn't easy to burst into laughter when you're about to burst with anger or tension. But that's not the idea. Laughter works when you use it to provide little outbursts of mirth so that stress never gets a chance to build up. Seek laughter therapy, not when you're distressed, but when you're already happy. On a day when you feel energetic and creative, take time to make room for more laughter in your life:

- Take some old issues of *Mad Magazine* to work. During your tea break, clip out the most giggle-inducing cartoons and put them up on your bulletin board or your door. Change them around often so that you aren't stuck with stale jokes that no longer evoke laughter.

- Tote along a fun photo frame to the office. Print out a funny quotation and tuck it into the frame. Place this at your desk to entertain yourself and others. (I've put up Robert Benchley's words — "A freelance writer is a man who is paid per piece, or per word, or perhaps" — to keep my sense of humor alive as I type those query letters by the dozen.) These days, you can buy "talking photo frames" that will let you record a joke or funny saying. This can be especially fun if you and a friend both have talking photo frames; you can sneak in and record new jokes on each other's frames so that they never get old.

- Surf the Internet for good, clean jokes — then mail a couple of them to your colleagues.

- You can start a humor file, into which you jot rib-tickling one-liners and jokes. When they start feeling stale, you can always give your file to a friend who's feeling blue.

- If you have a few moments to yourself, think back to a really funny incident from your life. Then entertain your colleagues with it at lunch. Instant popularity, too!

- When you go to the library, stop by the humor section and borrow a hilarious book or movie.

- Do your visits to the bookstore always follow the same pattern: Head for "Religion and Philosophy" or "Fiction," grab a latte, settle down for two hours, move out? Next time, take a detour: Spend a few minutes in the humor section. You'll find it refreshing.

- Keep comic books by your bedside.

- Create a comic-book-filled "basket of laughter" by the fireplace. On snowy evenings, cozy up in a rocking chair with cocoa and kids, and laugh the evening away.

- Change the message on your answering machine to an upbeat, humorous one.

- Give playful captions to your family photographs.

- Learn to laugh at yourself. If your stress has caused you

to be less than friendly, organized, or creative lately, explain your behavior to your colleagues or family with a fun quote on a placard, such as the often-quoted anonymous poem:

> *Roses are red,*
> *Violets are blue;*
> *I'm schizophrenic,*
> *And so am I.*

Lighten up. You'll brighten up.

Feel Better with Verse

LET'S FACE IT, sometimes fun and laughter feel just "too chipper" for comfort when you're stressed. Does this mean you should delve into a depressing piece of literature? Yes and no.

Experts say that reading a poignant, emotional poem when you're feeling low is actually a good idea because it "agrees" with your mood at the time. However, do choose verse that has a note of optimism and hope — a comforting, positive one. Mihaly Csikszentmihalyi, Ph.D., author of several books on creativity, said, "Sometimes, even one word is enough to open a window on a new view of the world, to start the mind on an inner journey." At the end of a tiring day, a poem can rock you into relaxation.

To find inspirational, healing poems, turn to poets such as Robert Bly, Rita Dove, or Elizabeth Barrett Browning, or look up recent Pulitzer Prize—winning poets on the Internet, for example, Maya Angelou. The following verse by Emily Dickinson is also quite uplifting:

> *"Hope" is the thing with feathers —*
> *That perches in the soul —*
> *And sings the song without the words —*
> *And never stops — at all —* [2]

If a poem stirs something in you, try to write or paint your emotions. Don't think you "can't write" or are "not an artist." Write from the heart, and the words will come. Let your pen or paintbrush move freely on the paper or canvas; the beauty of your own creation might take you by surprise.

Beat the Blues with Jazz

A MELODY FLOATING through the air is unseen, intangible. And yet it triggers a definite, concrete response in the human body. In rhythm with the melody, we start to release "happy chemicals" called endorphins, which have a profoundly healing effect on the mind. That is why spiritual teachers such as Dr. Deepak Chopra are collaborating with musicians to create music that heals. (As I write this, I'm listening to light, fluid tunes from *The Magic of Healing Music,* an album created by Bruce BecVar for Dr. Chopra.)

While Western music is generally designed to build to a crescendo then bring release, "new age" or spiritual music doesn't have a frenzied feeling; it is slow and gentle. So when you're in the mood for relaxation, listen to laid-back notes; they heal.

I remember a cold, rainy evening when I was in a mood as gray as the weather. On impulse, I went out for a drive. For a while I listened to a CD, but even that didn't help; I was just too restless. Suddenly, I knew what to do. I rolled up the windows, switched off the CD, and began to sing — first softly, then boldly. What came out wasn't Celine Dion, but the simple act of opening my lungs and my heart and singing for my own pleasure was immensely therapeutic. I returned home humming.

To me, music isn't simply about listening to songs or singing them. It is about creating harmony in your living spaces. Take alarm clocks: Aren't they the very antithesis of harmony? Do you relish their harsh trrrring or persistent beep in the morning? To me, those sounds feel shocking, as if I've jumped straight out of bed into a lake of icy water. An excellent way to set the tone for a lovely day is to buy an alarm clock that wakes you up to a sweet melody, or the gentle sound of wind chimes, or a simple bird song. Then stretch, like a satisfied cat on a lazy afternoon. Savor the pleasure of lying in bed just a minute or two before you plunge into another day.

Incidentally, a poll on the popular Website www.wordsmith.com revealed that "mellifluous," which means "sweet-sounding," is the most loved word in the English language.

When All Else Fails, Give Thanks

SOMETIMES LIFE seems so unfair that you can't stop asking, "Why me?" "Why this?" "Why now?" Usually there are no satisfactory answers to these questions, and nothing seems to be able to pull you out of the depths of depression. When that happens, turn inward and become your own source of solace.

Breathe deeply and give thanks for being alive. Feel grateful to have the use of your limbs and vital organs. Say "happy me, lucky me" — even if you feel exactly the opposite of happy and lucky. Say, "I am thankful..."

- For the tax returns I have to file, because it means that I am employed.

- For the mess I have to clean up after the party, because it means that I have the gift of friends.

- For a floor that needs mopping and windows that need cleaning, because it means I have a home.

- For this difficult situation, because it is an opportunity for me to make a wise decision and emerge stronger.

In her book *Undress Your Stress,* Lois Levy reminds us to "stop and give thanks whenever we are feeling low."[3] Be grateful for something. — one thing. I don't care what it is: eyesight, sunshine, ice cream, e-mail, breathing. Try it; it works.

Let me leave you with some healing thoughts on Aikido, a Japanese martial art that teaches harmony. Kicks, punches...and harmony? Sounds paradoxical, doesn't it? But the explanation is beautiful: An Aikido master moves to protect not only himself but also his attacker, redirecting the latter's energy so that he loses the desire to fight.

The Aikido principle, I think, can be more than a martial art; it can be a way of life. Without donning a uniform or lifting a leg to kick out, we can learn to beat back stress — an enemy that torments us all. How? The key is that Aikido teaches gentleness and compassion. It helps you mobilize your energies in such a way that you empathize with the enemy; you begin to understand why an unpleasant situation has arisen. And to understand, said a wise sage, is to forgive.

To bring home this point, let me tell you the story of Lord Buddha and the drunken elephant. Legend says that Lord Buddha's cousin, Devadatta, felt extremely jealous of the Buddha's rising popularity and plotted to kill him on several occasions. Once he forced an elephant to drink alcohol, beat it until it was crazed with anger, then let it loose toward the Buddha. Everyone around the Buddha ran away in panic, but the Buddha, seeing this drunken, crazed animal, felt nothing but pity and love for the creature. So strong was this feeling that the raging elephant could feel its power. To the amazement of all, the elephant stopped charging and lay down humbly at the Buddha's feet.

Fast-forwarding many centuries to the present day, I understand that it takes far less than a raging elephant to throw us into a state of panic. But if we remind ourselves that we're all blessed with the ability to understand and forgive, we'll be able to deal much better with the fiercest of stresses.

I wish you peace.

THOUGHTS FROM LYNN SMITH,
INTERVENTIONIST FOR
COLLEGE STUDENTS, 40

I am a very blessed individual who has had a fulfilling and purpose-driven life. I work outside of the home as an interventionist for college students, performing a form of counseling called Motivational Interviewing. Our main focus is the drinking habits of eighteen to twenty-four year olds, helping them to see how their habits can negatively affect their lives. My passion is to make a difference in someone's life each day, and this job allows me to do just that. Since I have such a rewarding and fulfilling career, I believe my stress level at work is kept to a minimum.

I am also a very busy mother and wife. My husband has an hour and a half commute each way to work. I try to take as much on as I possibly can family-wise, so he doesn't have to. With that said, I am the one who worries about each person's appointments, school functions, extracurricular activities, and social schedule as well as the general running of the home. I may be blessed in the limited amount of stress in my career but the stress for the home life and trying to juggle both a career and loving family life more than makes up for it.

Normally, my time to de-stress is after the family is in bed. That's the only period of time I have to reflect on myself, my day, and my life. The one thing that allows me to have the most inner peace is to brew a pot of naturally organic loose tea, it's called comfort tea. It's a wonderfully sweet aromatic, spearmint type tea. As soon as I smell the minty aroma, my troubles instantly begin to melt. I am a candle person and have several different types of aromatic groupings through out my home. To add to my calming environment I love to light a few, smell the aroma, and watch the flames flicker. I put on CDs that are instrumental, such a George Winston (piano) or Kenny G (jazz). These add to my calming environment. This de-stress time allows me to get "my house" in order. I try hard to have a clean and organized home for my family and have noticed over the years that, more importantly, my personal "spiritual house" has to be in order so that I can be the best person possible for all those around me.

These things together allow me to reflect on all the wonderful gifts and joys of my life. Once I begin to realize just how much I have, my stresses just don't seem to be important anymore and slowly disappear. I have always felt that attitude about life is very important and once I have complete control over that, then I can face even the hardest situations with a smile, and the faith that the problems really aren't problems after all.

Chapter Summary and Resources

- Life's small discomforts can add up to create big stress. Don't let stress build up!

- Cut down on your commitments.

- Don't procrastinate. To help you do this, there's a popular Website, www.flylady.com; the everyday wisdom you'll find there will help you do your chores in a systematic and organized manner.

- Make life comfortable. Shop for essential items that make daily living easier. Good starting points: Home Depot, the Container Store, or even the yard sales in your neighborhood.

- Tame the time monster. Ask friends to share their successful time-management tips. Attend a workshop on the subject of managing time. Visit www.stresstips.com for scores of resources on dealing with various aspects of stress.

- Calm stress with good nutrition.

- Rub stress away with a healing massage. A good book to read is *Instant Calm: Over 100 Easy-to-Use Techniques For Relaxing Mind and Body,* by Paul Wilson (Plume, 1999).

- Smile. The moment you smile, you start to heal. For inspiration, read *All Smiles,* edited by Bruce Velick — a feel-good book that features smiling people from all over the world (Chronicle Books, 1995).

- Get close to someone. Catch up with a friend and go out to the movies. Think about joining a group where you'll meet people. "The Art of Living" is one such class. Inspired by the teachings of spiritual master Sri Sri Ravishankar, the Art of Living Foundation is a non-profit organization that aims to eliminate the effects of stress from your system. The six-day Art of Living workshop promises: "More energy, more clarity, more love, more happiness, more celebration, more depth, more silence." Offered in more than 140 countries, there is sure to be a course near where you live. For more information, visit www.artofliving.com.

- Laugh. It really is the best medicine! In addition to the gentle jokes in *Reader's Digest,* you can find a treasure house of laughs on Websites such as www.cleanjokes.net and www.ahajokes.com.

- Heal with art.

- Give thanks.

CHAPTER 7

Bliss

How to Be Simply, Spiritually Happy

*I have the pleasure of a passing moment —
and what more can a mortal ask?*

— GEORGE GISSING

Gentle fingers knead my back, laving it with warm oil.
Bliss. Slowly, softly, pleasure diffuses through my being,
like cream dissolving into cappuccino. In this moment, I
know that pure bliss is simple. It is free. And wherever you are,
however busy, you can always find a few moments of bliss.

I'm so glad I allowed myself to enjoy this fifteen-minute chair
massage at the mall — free of charge and purely on impulse.

Fill This Moment; It Is Bliss

HOW IS YOUR DAY GOING? Or is it going, going, gone — just like
that, in the blink of an eye? Is the roller coaster of your life running
so fast you're afraid to jump off? If so, let me tell you a beautiful
Zen story from Japan:

> *A man was being chased across a field by a ferocious tiger.*
> *At the edge of the field, there was a cliff. To escape the tiger,*

the man caught hold of a vine and swung himself over the edge of the cliff. Dangling down, he saw that there were more tigers on the ground below him! To make matters worse, two mice were gnawing at the vine to which he clung. He knew that at any moment, he would fall to certain death. That's when he noticed a wild strawberry growing on the cliff wall. Clutching the vine with one hand, he plucked the strawberry with the other and put it in his mouth.

He had never before realized how sweet a strawberry could taste.

What a poignant message! Life offers hundreds of simple pleasures, as sweet as the taste of a strawberry. They're yours for the taking, yours for free. Seize them! Don't postpone until tomorrow — or even the next hour — what you can enjoy today, at this moment.

Let me suggest some succulent ways to slow down and savor the moment:

- Sit in your backyard or bay window, sketching a tree, reading a book, or just daydreaming.

- Dance to "The Time of My Life" — even if you have two left feet.

- Listen to the love theme from *Out of Africa* with your sweetheart on a moonlit night. Or pump up the volume and enjoy a zesty old favorite.

- Watch the first redwings of spring splash and dip in your birdbath.

- Soak in the many moods of a tree: thoughtful in its stillness, swaying in the wild wind like a fan at a rock concert, looking radiant after a rain bath.

- Enjoy India-style corn next time you have a rainstorm. At monsoon, the bazaars of India come alive with the aroma of corn roasted over hot coals. Rub roasted ears of corn with slices of lemon dipped in a mixture of rock salt and black pepper. Pull a chair up to your window and mmmunch to the sound of the pouring rain. The lemony juice might dribble down your chin, but that is as it should be!

- Savor the aroma of grilled onion and peppers on a summer afternoon.

- Chat with your best friend over chai tea, hot scones, and homemade jam. (See the sidebar on pages 182–84 for fragrant chai recipes.)

- Take off your shoes, then flop like a rag doll on your bed for a long time after a hard day.

- Wake up your skin and senses with a refreshing rosewater spritz at the end of a long day. Organic rosewater, made from fresh, bug-free petals, not only heals and refreshes all types of skin, but also suffuses your senses with its lingering fragrance.

THEN THERE ARE little bliss-breaks that, while being equally simple, are refreshingly different. Here are some terrific ideas I've come across:

Smile with Your Whole Being

FLIP THROUGH A FAMILY ALBUM, watch your wedding video, or just close your eyes and think back to a time when you were truly happy. Remember the day at the beach when you built sand castles with your kids, a vacation when you reconnected with your spouse, or the day you spent in your pajamas reading an enchanting book. Sweet memories always make you smile. When you feel the smile coming, envision it seeping through your whole being, from the tips of your toes, across your heart, to the top of your head, into every cell.

CHAI RECIPES: BREW UP SOME BLISS

Simple, Soothing Chai

1 cup water

1 cup milk

2 teaspoons sugar

2 teaspoons black tea leaves

1 pod green cardamom, crushed

1/4-inch piece of fresh ginger root, peeled

To make fragrant chai as it is enjoyed in India, boil the water with the milk. As the bubbles rise to the surface, drop in the sugar, tea, cardamom, and ginger. Reduce the heat and turn it up again repeatedly to allow the chai to come to three or four boils. Then strain and enjoy two steaming cups of bliss or share one with a friend.

Spice-Spiked Chai for a Rainy Afternoon

This recipe is a great perk-up treat on a damp day. Also, the "hot" spices in this chai are wonderful for clearing out phlegm and mucus, so it's an ideal brew to concoct when you're suffering from a cold.

2 whole cloves

1 green cardamom pod

1/2 cinnamon stick, broken into pieces

1¹/₂ cups water

¹/₄ teaspoon ground ginger root

¹/₈ teaspoon freshly ground black pepper

¹/₂ cup milk

2 tablespoons granulated sugar

2 tablespoons black tea leaves (Darjeeling tea is great)

Crush the cloves, cardamom, and cinnamon, using a mortar and pestle or a clean coffee grinder. Transfer the crushed spices into a medium-sized pan, then pour in the water. Add the ginger and pepper and bring it to a boil.

Remove the pan from the heat, cover, and let it steep for about five minutes. Now pour in the milk, stir the sugar into the brew, and set the pan on the stove again. When the mixture boils, remove the pan from heat and stir in the tea leaves. Cover and steep for another three minutes or so. Stir the chai, then strain and serve it piping hot. Serves two.

Mild-and-Mellow Cardamom Chai For a Laid-Back Morning

In India, traditional healers consider cardamom to be a cooling spice, so this tea is ideal for days when you're feeling in need of some mind-body comfort.

2¹/₂ cups water

1 cup milk

2 green cardamom pods, split open, seeds intact

4 teaspoons granulated sugar

2 teaspoons green tea leaves

Combine water, sugar, and milk in a medium-sized pan, and bring them to a boil. Remove the pan from heat, add the cardamom pods, and steep for about three minutes, uncovered. Add the tea leaves, stir lightly, and let sit for two more minutes, still uncovered. Strain and sip. Serves two.

Hot Idea!

Next time you brew chai, don't restrict yourself to cardamom and cinnamon. Spice up your tea with chocolate, vanilla beans, licorice root, nutmeg, coriander...you'll be surprised at the number of happy companions tea can take!

Excerpt From My Journal:

Darjeeling, India, July, 1989

It rained last night, and it was as if all of nature had made tea. Warm leaves suddenly brewed a bit of their surface essence, sending their scent wafting through the window. Dar-jeeling...this is nature's teapot. How I love to stand atop a peak and watch the endless carpet of tea — hill after hill after hill. After a while, the high energy of the place starts to hum in my ears. Billions upon billions of tea leaves are being born here. Six inches above the tea leaves, everything is shimmering, like a mirage. To think that tea is taken to be a light drink, whereas it's made of so much healing energy from the earth and the sun.

Touch a "Marma" Point on Your Body

THE WORD MARMA means "hidden" or "secret." You have 107 "secret" points — places on your body where two or more types of tissue meet. Ayurvedic healers describe the marmas as "bridges between your physical and spiritual energies." So pressing a marma point is an exquisite feeling. Here are three easy-to-locate marma points on your body:

- the hollow of your temples, on either side of your head
- the sides of your nose where your nostrils flare

- the center of your wrist, just below your hand (palm facing up)

To energize your marmas, place a few drops of warm sesame or almond oil on your fingertips, then rub the area gently for a minute or two. Breathe gently and deeply as you do this. Brew a cup of healing chamomile tea, and enjoy it afterward.

Rejuvenate Your "Rasa"

RASA, IN SANSKRIT, is the essence or "juice" of life. The healers of India believe that when we're young, we're rich with rasa: The skin is moist, digestion is efficient, and energy levels are at their peak. As we grow older, our reserves of essential energy become depleted, resulting in low vitality, poor health, and that "over the hill" feeling.

Restoring your rasa can be a joyous journey — and it needn't be a long, tiring one, either. Just for a day, commit yourself to conserving your energy for things you really enjoy. Here are some ideas on how you can do this:

- Eat lightly throughout the day. Heavy meals place great stress on the body's digestive system, draining you of rasa.

- Eat foods that actually replenish your rasa; these are called rasayanas (rasa: juice, ayana: bring in). Fresh, organic fruits and vegetables, light soups and salads, whole grains, nuts (particularly almonds), and organic yogurt — all of these qualify as rasayanas.

- Give your overworked senses a reprieve. If you were planning to work on the computer for three hours, work for one hour instead. Then take a break and come back to your desk later — if you feel like it. Otherwise, take half the day off and spend it in the comfort of your home. Similarly, cut down — just for the day — on Internet surfing and television watching, which strain your eyes, back, and brain.

• Take a healing nap; it's the easiest, most pleasurable way to conserve your rasa. Sleep researchers have found that a "power nap" can work as a mini-hibernation, reversing information overload and helping you think better. If you can't afford to take a fifteen-minute nap in bed, simply put your head down on your desk and close your eyes for a few minutes. You'll wake up with energy to burn.

• Get into bed a little early. Prepare for bedtime like you would for a date (bedtime can be a wonderful way to date yourself!): Take a warm shower, pamper your skin with a softening after-bath lotion, dim the lights, and climb into the comfort of crisp, clean sheets. Surround yourself with sights and sounds that say "serenity": incense, a sprig of lavender, or scented candles (take care: never leave a burning candle unattended); wind chimes, a soothing CD, a water fountain, or a hand-crafted wooden flute; crystals, seashells, or artwork that relaxes you; crisp air flowing in through an open window. Breathe deeply, and let your mind gradually settle into restfulness. This night of restful sleep will endow you with a bounty of rasa for the next day.

Dream

"HOLD FAST YOUR DREAMS!/Within your heart/Keep one still, secret spot/Where dreams may go,"[1] wrote Louise Driscoll. A dream can be anything from an expression of your deepest desires to a declaration of great intent. Tuck little "journals of dreams" by your bedside, in your office drawer, or in your car. Big, small, sweet, silly, vague, concrete — let those pages hold all sorts of dreams you've had over the years. (I think journals make the best companions; every woman should give herself one!)

If you aren't passionate about writing, express yourself in a way that appeals to you:

- Sketch your dream. Paint it. Color it. Frame it.

- Say it on camera: Use a small video camera to make a movie about your dream.

- Sing your dream out loud. Do this as you take a shower; don't worry about reason or rhyme, just take the theme "My Dream," and let the words come pouring out.

Make Someone Else's Day

RESEARCH SHOWS that a simple act of kindness can work wonders for the way you feel. Allan Luks, author of *The Healing Power of Doing Good: The Health and Spiritual Benefits of Helping Others,* surveyed more than 3,000 volunteers of all ages across the country, asking them how they felt after doing a good deed. The results established that, after performing a kind act, most people feel a rush of euphoria, followed by a longer period of calm. Luks called this feeling "helper's high," and concluded that the initial rush of joy slowly gives way to long-lasting feelings of emotional well-being.[2]

Even if you're overstretched and don't have time to do someone a favor, you can make people around you happy through simple gestures and words. Smile at the next person you see. Give someone a pat or a hug. Be generous with compliments. Say a kind word. Some of the most beautiful phrases in the English language are:

- "You look beautiful."

- "I'm here for you."

- "Here is a little something for you."

- "I love you."

For ideas on other simple pleasures, turn to the book *Feel Good*, by Pamela Allardice (Allen & Unwin, 2001), or savor Jennifer Louden's evergreen companion, *The Woman's Comfort Book* (Harper, 1992).

More Blissful Books for Your Bedside

CRAWLING INTO A SNUG, warm bed on a chilly evening is a great source of bliss in itself. But if you're also reading a truly heart-warming book...ah! Of course, nothing quite matches the guilty pleasure of reading a whodunit or a romance, but from time to time treat your soul to a morsel of true bliss: Read a book that reminds you how beautiful life is — how precious, how worthy of being lived simply and mindfully.

For instance, I can never forget the evening I spent with Jon Kabat-Zinn through his book *Wherever You Go, There You Are: Mindfulness Meditation in Everyday Life*. He writes, "Dwelling inwardly for extended periods of time, we come to know something of the poverty of always looking outside of ourselves for happiness, understanding, and wisdom."[3]

Another author I tremendously enjoy is Nobel laureate Rabindranath Tagore. Life, hope, and joy sing in Tagore's poems through simple images of birds, flowers, clouds, and sunshine. Some of my favorite words from Tagore:

> Do not say, "It is morning," and dismiss it with a name
> of yesterday. See it for the first time as a newborn child that
> has no name.
>
> The butterfly counts not months but moments, and has time
> enough.
>
> The fish in the water is silent, the animal on the earth is noisy,

the bird in the air is singing. But man has in him the silence
of the sea, the noise of the earth, and the music of the air.[4]

Spend a blissful evening in a bookstore, browsing for books that promise to heal you. Then bring one home and let those tranquil pages lull you into a night of restfulness. (See Chapter Summary and Resources for other recommended reading.)

The Easiest Route to Bliss

SO FAR, we've talked about harnessing outward stimuli to create inner bliss. But there's a powerhouse of pleasures within your own being, waiting for you to discover them and make them your own. Let me begin with one such pleasure you can give yourself easily — any time, anywhere, and for free. Holding your breath with curiosity? Well, relax and breathe deeply. For that blissful secret is just that: learning to breathe — really breathe, not simply inhaling and exhaling through your nostrils, but breathing in and out with your lungs, your belly, and your whole being.

S-l-o-w Breathing is Blissful Because...

BIOLOGICALLY, deep breathing increases oxygen supply to the body's tissues and cells. Also, the act of breathing from the diaphragm "massages" our vital organs — the liver, heart, and stomach — promoting better circulation and a sense of alertness.

Spiritually, breath is seen as the thread that connects us with the world. The ancients called it prana — which, in Sanskrit, means "vitality," or life itself. We don't usually think of it this way, but sages who lived in India long ago said, "With every deep breath you take, you're inhaling more vitality, more prana."

Breathe Like a Yogi

IF YOU OBSERVE A YOGI, a Zen master, or a martial art trainer practicing meditation or exercise, you will notice that they always begin by drawing in a deep, deep breath.

Breathing is, in fact, seen as such a healing activity that yoga gurus have devised dozens of techniques for breathing correctly; some of them can seem quite complex. But it is the simplest yogic breathing that I find the most pleasurable and effective for day-to-day release and rejuvenation. It's called *naadi shodhana* ("naadi" means "channel," and "shodhana" means "to cleanse").

This is how you do it:

1. Gently press two fingers of your right hand against your left nostril to close it. Inhale slowly, deeply, and fully through your right nostril.

2. Now press your right thumb against your right nostril, and exhale through your left nostril — again, slowly, deeply, and fully.

3. Repeat, beginning with the left nostril this time.

There! You've just completed one full circuit of yogic breathing. Try it five to ten times, and feel yourself heal. This kind of breathing has helped me on many occasions: when I feel anger or resentment building up over a trivial matter, before a crucial meeting, or while flying in an airplane.

Breathe Positive

YOU CAN ALSO use your moments of deep breathing to make some simple, blissful affirmations. With every breath, you can say to yourself:

- "I'm inhaling vitality and exhaling fatigue."
- "I'm inhaling serenity and exhaling stress."
- "I'm inhaling love and exhaling anger."

SURROUND YOURSELF WITH SERENITY

Simple ways to bring a sense of calm to your environment:

At Work

- Use a soothing nature screensaver on your computer.

- Have plants such as ficus, palm, and spider plant in your office; they require little care, soothe the mind, and reduce indoor air pollution.

- Don't let your office look like a platter for spaghetti-like twines of wires and cables. Tie the cables up and tuck them behind the desk. Wherever the eye travels, let it find clean, uncluttered spaces.

- If you have space for it, place a small indoor fountain in your office; it will keep you calm throughout the day.

In the Garden

- Trim overgrown bushes.

- Create a pleasing, wide entryway to your home.

- Remove dead plants and replace them with fresh ones.

- Keep your yard free of debris.

- Plant only as many flower beds and bushes as you can easily tend.

- Fill your garden with colors that please you.

Inside Your Home

- Use soft lighting.

- Keep the thermostat at a comfortable temperature.

- Play soft music or soothing sounds.

- Use cool, calming colors.

- Put up healing decorations, such as a plant or a bunch of fresh flowers.

- Use aromatherapy candles, potpourri, flowers.

Remember to Breathe

OFTEN, THE PROBLEM isn't whether we know that we should breathe better; it's remembering to slow down and breathe deeply. Here are some easy ways to remind yourself:

- Set your watch to beep at regular — say, one-hour — intervals. Each time the beep sounds, stop whatever you are doing and start breathing deeply.

- When you wake up in the morning, set yourself some better-breathing cues. One day, you could choose a "just-before" rhythm: just before lunch, just before dinner, just before getting out of bed. The next day, try out "just-after" — just for fun and variety.

- If you're too busy to remember even your reminders, breathe deeply at bedtime. Even a few minutes can be very relaxing; as a bonus, you'll sleep better.

Deeper Bliss

TO MAKE BLISS a part of your life — to soak it in so deeply that it becomes YOU — combine your practice of deep breathing with mindful meditation. It isn't difficult at all. Basically, all you're doing is becoming completely present in the moment as you breathe. Spiritual teachers call this "mindfulness."

The Meaning of Mindfulness

I LOVE THESE TWO oft-quoted tales about the Buddha; they capture the essence of mindful living:

> One day, the Buddha was taking a walk with his disciple, Ananda. They were absorbed in a deeply spiritual discussion. Just then, a fly came and perched itself on the Buddha's

face. His hand flew up to brush the fly away. Then, after a moment, the Buddha repeated the action of brushing it away. Puzzled, Ananda asked him, "Why did you repeat your action, even though the fly is no longer on your face?" The Buddha replied, "The first time, I brushed the fly away absently, automatically. This time, I wanted to bring awareness to my action."

Another time, someone asked the Buddha, "What do you do?" He replied, "I walk, I eat, I sleep." The questioner asked, "What is so special about that? We all do the same things." The Buddha replied, "Yes, but when I walk, I really walk. When I eat, I really eat. And when I sleep, I really sleep."

This, then, is the key: to stop living in the future ("I've got to do the dishes quickly, so I can reach my yoga class on time") or the past (sitting in a movie theater, thinking, "How did I forget to renew my license?"). Whether you are sitting, walking, kneading dough, ironing clothes, driving, working at the computer, or eating dinner, being present in the moment is the secret of living life to the fullest.

What Happens When You Sit Still?

LET US LOOK at the simple act of sitting still; no other activity illustrates how restless we really are. The "monkey mind" starts chattering louder and faster than ever. Thoughts, worries, fears, regrets, questions, doubts — all of these tumble inside your brain and tangle your nerves. Why? Because we are afraid to sit still. We're afraid to allow ourselves to be present in our stillness. We are more comfortable with worrying, hurrying, doing something. But it is possible to relax while "doing nothing." Next time you sit still:

- Don't fight your thoughts. Think of them as strangers you pass on the street. Like you, they're strolling by; they're not friends, they're not foes, they're just part of the normal flow of life.

- Don't try to chant a mantra.

- Don't focus on a thought or object.

- Don't contemplate the meaning of life.

Simply sit in a comfortable position, and allow your body and your mind to take a rest. Close your eyes if you like, or keep them open. Slowly, you will become aware of the warm, slow breath that enters and leaves your being. Your limbs will feel loose, limp, and wonderfully relaxed. Your mind will feel soothed and settled, in spite of the thoughts still flowing through it.

Rejoice! You have just experienced the pure bliss of being present in the moment. Call it mindfulness, call it meditation — it works! Here is an excerpt from my journal on the day when I experienced this exquisite feeling for the first time:

> *I can best describe it as euphoria: a clear, deep feeling of happiness, a cheerful bubble of bliss that rose to the surface of my heart. There was no thought in my mind, no obstruction, nothing but happiness. I don't think the feeling lasted beyond a few seconds, but in those moments I touched the core of my being. I felt my soul.*

The yogis of India even have a Sanskrit name for this delicious feeling; they call it samadhi, or "the fourth state of consciousness" — a state superior to the other three that we ordinarily experience: sleep, wakefulness, and dreaming.

The Magic of Meditation

ONE THING IS FOR SURE: Meditation can be an antidote for any kind of stress. The very meaning of the word "meditation" is rooted in the Latin *meditatus,* which means "to remedy." Modern research has shown the profound health benefits of meditation. Here are the basics at a glance:

- Your pulse rate slows down.

- Your blood pressure becomes lower.

- Your muscles relax.

- Your nervous system begins to function more calmly.

- Your body stops producing plasma cortisol, a stress hormone.

And that's just for starters!

The more you meditate, the easier it becomes for you to relax in a tense situation. You become more tuned in to your emotions and, as a result, you are better able to understand the desires and emotions of others. Life's edges become softer — and sweeter.

Several years ago, when I was based in Delhi, India's capital city, I signed up for a five-day meditation class — and it changed my life. I cannot resist sharing with you the story of how I chanced upon bliss.

I Tried Meditation

A BIT OF BACKGROUND may help. I'm a perfectly normal big-city gal with a normal big-city job at a glamorous women's magazine. In other words, my days dissolve into one another in a dizzying cycle of writing punch lines, meeting deadlines, chopping words, hopping events, meeting people, and, in the process, conveniently forgetting all about myself.

Now picture this perfectly normal gal on a perfectly blue Monday morning. We're at the monthly editorial meeting, feeling exactly like lambs about to be sacrificed. I am rummaging desperately in the cupboards of my mind for crumbs of ideas for articles. Several not-so-inspiring ideas bob in: how to be a smart shopper, how to impress your boss, how to be a sensible health nut, what you should never say at an interview...

But today, the editor doesn't ask us to reel off our ideas. Instead, she has a gleam in her eye that suggests she's come up with some ideas of her own... very dangerous. It's funny how all of us are suddenly concentrating firmly on our shoes.

The boss says she wants an article on meditation. "It's the in thing," she gushes. "Celebrities are doing it. Businesses are giving their employees time off to take the five-day course. Why doesn't one of you find out about meditation? I believe they teach a popular meditation technique here in Delhi. It'll make a zesty four-pager."

There's an uncomfortable, heads-down silence.

Then I make the mistake of looking up at my boss — and the story is mine.

Back at my desk, I sigh: 2,500 words to generate and two weeks to generate them in! I'm wondering where to begin, when my boss leans over my desk: "Here, this could be a good starting point for you." It's a phone number.

I call the number and a polite voice responds. I ask about the meditation course, and the soft-spoken gentleman tells me I'm in luck: I can join the five-day course next Monday evening. He proceeds to give me the course schedule.

I am about to say that I only want information from the meditation teacher for my article, but I stop myself just in time. It suddenly strikes me as a good idea to attend the whole course. I know that my article will shape up beautifully if I do it in the first person. Why reveal to them who I am, and end up with a rah-rah report that may or may not be true? So I pretend to be a new meditation enthusiast, and I promise to be there at 6:00 P.M. on Monday.

Day One at the Meditation Center

THE TEACHER, tall and lean, looks like he has just emerged from a bath. His all-white clothes are bright as freshly fallen snow, and his generous beard looks good on him. In fact, he has the looks of a typical mantra-chanting, prayer-performing, sermon-preaching mendicant. He smiles around at us.

"A very warm welcome to you, friends," he begins. His voice is crisp and compelling. "I am happy to be initiating you into the practice of meditation. It is a natural, effortless process that allows the mind to experience subtler and subtler levels of the thinking process until thinking is transcended and the mind comes into direct contact with the source of thought."

He continues, "You might wonder what I mean by 'the source of thought.' Let me explain: Just like a bubble of water is formed on the floor of the ocean before it rises to the surface, your thoughts are born deep inside your mind, in a place where there is nothing but pure energy. That is the source of your thought. At its source, all thought is born pure and uncorrupted. But as it bubbles up to the surface, it gets mutilated by the negative emotions and stresses along the way.

"If you can somehow reach out to that source and let your thoughts rise up to the surface of your mind undefiled by stress or negativity, you can actually change the way you think, feel, and live. Meditation promises to help you unlock that infinite potential inside you."

Now the teacher adds something surprising. He tells us this meditation technique is so easy that children can learn it in just four days, while adults take five. That's because children are unprejudiced, with no preconceived ideas about meditation, while we adults need that extra day to "unlearn" a few things. Interesting.

Day Two

ONE BY ONE, the teacher whispers a word in each of our ears. It is not even a word, actually — just a two-syllable sound. He calls it a mantra, and instructs us not to share it with anyone, not even our spouse.

Once we all have our mantras, the teacher says, "We shall now meditate for twenty minutes." Just like that. No further instructions on what to do with the mantra. Repeat it, I assume.

Here we go.

I am sitting, eyes closed. I can never get the lotus position right, so I just tuck my legs up under myself and get comfortable. I can hear the soft sounds of breathing around me. Someone moves furniture upstairs. Someone in the room coughs.

I silently chant the mantra...slowly...once, twice, three times, and then...a thought floats in — an awful one, at that. I suddenly remember that I promised my editor a one-page filler on "Dating Dos and Don'ts" by tomorrow morning — and I haven't even started it! I just clean forgot. Oh, dear.

I hastily remind myself of the mantra, and start chanting again. Once, twice, three times, four times, and then...here comes another thought: the India-Pakistan cricket match, this time. It's going to be a cliffhanger — but, hey, why am I thinking about something as frivolous as a cricket match when I ought to be chanting? I pull myself back to the mantra, this time with more success. I think it's been about five minutes, and guess what? I'm starting to feel...sleepy!

Yes, I can feel myself dozing off. My eyes are getting deliciously heavy. The mantra recedes to the back of my mind, while I shamelessly enjoy a brief nap.

The teacher's crisp voice floats into the silence, asking us to open our eyes slowly. A few moments of silence, then he asks gently, "Did you feel sleepy at any time during the meditation?"

Yes, everyone admits sheepishly that they've been sleeping. The teacher's reaction is quite surprising. "Good," he says. "That was a little of your pent-up stress escaping — the body and the mind catching up on much-needed rest. You closed your eyes and slipped into a state of quietude. There were no sounds in the room except soft breathing. The atmosphere allowed your mind to bring the superficial stresses bubbling up to the surface and free them into space. It lightened you up."

With that, we disperse for the evening, with instructions to practice meditation at home in the morning.

Day Three

I'M UP EARLY. A bath and a bowl of cornflakes later, I am in my study, door closed, eyes closed. The family has been warned not to disturb me. The first five minutes are wonderful. I manage my mantra-chanting very well.

Automatically, I fall into the rhythm of chanting. I'm beginning to feel very glad, when cruel knuckles pound on the door. My eyes fly open, and I fly into one of my darkest rages. It's the phone — what else? They couldn't say I didn't want to be disturbed, because it was the boss herself on the line, wanting to know how it went. "Well, it's gone," I want to yell. And it is. I leave home in a perfectly terrible mood, leaving my glass of juice to sulk on the table.

So much for bliss.

On my way to work, I'm still fuming about my failed attempt at bliss: angry with my family for not letting me be, disappointed in myself for losing my temper. Then it strikes me: Didn't the teacher promise that this form of meditation is not about concentrating? Then why are we chanting this mantra? I'm suddenly indignant — and angry. I can't wait to ask him for an explanation.

Back to the meditation center after a long, hard day. I'm wondering how to confess that I couldn't do it, but I find out that many others are in the same boat. At least five others in the group have not been able to meditate at all: One got stuck in a traffic jam, another had unexpected guests, a third had a headache, and so on. I realize that I actually seem to have done better than most: five full minutes!

The teacher tackles all our grumbling with his usual calm demeanor. A few assurances later, I burst out with the question that's been nagging me: Why are we concentrating?

The teacher, unruffled, asks a question in return: "Why are you concentrating?"

I'm speechless.

Yes, come to think of it, he never did ask us to concentrate, did he?

He smiles: "It is natural to try to concentrate, because that's how we are conditioned to meditate. But next time you practice, don't worry about being disturbed. Let the phone ring, let people bang on the door. Just open your eyes and gently signal them to wait. If it is something that demands your immediate attention, go and attend to it. Then come back and go into silence once again."

It's as if the fog has suddenly cleared from my eyes.

The next two days were blissful. We sat together in meditation, and compared notes and shared our experiences afterward.

SO THIS IS MEDITATION: the freedom to think, feel, dream — without restriction, without interference. I cannot say it better than the teacher, who asked us to imagine the mind to be a glass of muddy water. "Shake it," he said, "And the mud will toss about in the glass.

Leave it alone, and it will gradually settle down, leaving the water clear right down to the bottom. Meditation is about learning to leave this glass alone."

And that is how I stumbled into meditation. Looking back, I am glad I didn't join those classes for the usual reasons: because I was stressed or because everyone else was doing it. I went into the classes full of questions and doubts, and I emerged more connected with myself than I had been for a long, long time.

Today, I begin my mornings and end my days by sitting still and allowing myself to do the simplest — and ironically, the toughest — thing a human being can do these days: just breathe, just be. I look forward to my meditation sessions like a child waits for a favorite cartoon show, or like an adult longs to walk barefoot on soft, moist grass. And, always, I emerge from meditation with a sense of having enjoyed a twenty-minute vacation — more refreshing than a full eight-hour night of sleep.

Teach Yourself Meditation

THOUGH I KNOW how wonderful the experience of learning meditation from a teacher is, I also understand that taking a course can be an added demand on your time and your pocketbook (I was fortunate to have learned it for free, but that was back in India when all they asked for was voluntary donations). If so, let a book, a video, or an audiotape put you on the road to tranquility at a fraction of the price you would pay for a course, and at your own leisure.

You can find some fabulous meditation resources at your public library. *Meditation for Beginners* is a DVD that I watched and enjoyed. Released in 2001 by Yoga Zone, this is an excellent, three-part introduction to meditation. It teaches you an easy yoga stretch, how to meditate by scanning your body, and how to refresh your mind with meditation.

Walking Meditation

IF THE IDEA of sitting in one place to meditate makes you feel restless, don't think that meditation isn't for you. Walking meditation is a fabulous alternative; think of it as meditation in action. Here's how it works:

- Put on a comfortable pair of walking shoes.

- Start walking.

- Walk slowly and naturally, letting your arms swing by your sides. As your feet touch the ground, say "step, step, step," or "one, two, three," or "left, right, left." This will help you focus on the act of walking, rather than allowing your thoughts to start "chattering" as is their wont.

- Then, when your feet connect with the earth beneath, your senses open up to the beauty that surrounds you, and your mind begins to feel centered, make up your own simple meditations as you go along. Have a gentle, life-affirming dialogue with your higher self.

Blissful Thoughts

LET ME LEAVE YOU with some meditative reflections from my personal journal:

> *This moment is mine.*
> *I have nothing to take away from this moment,*
> *nothing to add to it.*
> *I am happy breathing out.*
> *I am happy breathing in.*
> *This moment is bliss.*

Today, I slow down to notice the beauty that surrounds me. It is everywhere: in the wrinkled smile of a grandmother, in the faithful eyes of my dog, in a blade of grass lit by the sun, in my own heart.

Beauty is not an illusion; it is not an endless quest. It is simple, and it resides in the here and the now and the everyday.

This beauty I discover anew is a source of joy.

Let my heart be lit with its glow.

Waves of joy wash over me as I think of my connection with the vast family of the universe. This earth beneath my feet is my anchor — the sky, my roof. The air I breathe is life itself. Sunshine gives me cheer. The ocean teaches me to be calm. With open arms, nature embraces me and assures me that I am happy, safe, and loved. With all its cares and worries, this world is a beautiful place, and I am fortunate to be part of it. I am thankful for my countless blessings.

Chapter Summary and Resources

- Life is short. Don't postpone pleasure.

- Each day brings you a chance to exult in the magic of life: birds, trees, sunshine, blue skies, food, friends. Give yourself permission to enjoy them all.

- Sweet memories make you smile. Once in a while, traipse down memory lane with cards, letters, and pictures you've gathered over the years.

- Ancient healers of India identified 107 "marma points" on the human body. These points, when gently massaged, soothe both body and mind.

- Imagine that you are a vessel filled with rasa, the fresh, sparkling juice of life. Don't let life's pressures drain your rasa away! The key to conserving rasa: make "everything in moderation" your mantra for life.

- Dreams drift you away from the cares of the world, even if for a short while, so it's essential to dream every now and then. Envision what you'd love to do most, and let the thought of it heal you.

- Do good. Be good. You'll love it. For inspiration, read *Gesundheit* (Inner Traditions International Limited, 1998), the touching, true-life story of Patch Adams, a doctor who gave healing an altogether new meaning with his personal touch. The book was the inspiration for a beautiful film called *Patch Adams,* starring Robin Williams as the doctor with the golden heart.

- Art is bliss. An uplifting work of fiction, a beautiful painting, a book of sayings, or a film that celebrates life — each of these has the potential to bring you tremendous calm and cheer. Here's a short list of my favorites:

  Movies

  1. *Titanic:* The lyrics of Celine Dion's beautiful song, "My Heart Will Go On," sit on this movie like a tea-cozy.

  2. *Ghost:* I've watched the scene where Patrick Swayze's ghost touches Demi Moore through Whoopi Goldberg's body so many times that my video cassette has begun automatically rewinding itself at the point where the song "Unchained Melody" ends!

3. *Amelie:* The endearing story of a little girl who craves love, *Amelie* is French cinema at its most magical. Amelie makes other people's happiness her goal in life, with soul-stirring results.

4. *Casablanca:* What can I say? Every time I watch it, the agony in Ingrid Bergman's eyes makes me cry, and Humphrey Bogart makes me fall in love with love all over again.

5. *Chocolat:* It's everything a feel-good movie should be: sensual, seductive, yet essentially simple. Juliette Binoche is superb as the chocolatier who teaches the folks of a French village to slow down and savor life.

Books

1. *The Greatest Salesman in the World,* by Og Mandino (Bantam Books, 1968): This is an inspiring little parable. On the face of it, it's a book about

ROSIBEL GUZMAN, MANAGING EDITOR, *AMERICAN FITNESS* MAGAZINE, 25

Simple things spell "bliss" for me: the scent of candles around me after a hard, stressful day; the sound of music while I shower; spending time with my loved ones — whether it is over a meal or going out to watch a movie — talking, laughing, and spending time with them does wonders to diminish my stress levels.

Water, in particular, is a blissful element in my life. After rushing all day, I take my time in the bath, enjoying the water and letting it relax me. Depending on my mood, I listen and sing along to soft, upbeat music or music with a strong message. And the simplest pleasure of them all: watching my favorite TV shows from the comfort of my couch.

making a sale. But its message is profound: Believe in yourself.

2. *The Greatest Gift,* by Philip Van Doren Stern (Penguin Books, 1996): The original story that inspired the Christmas classic *It's a Wonderful Life.* It's a simple, short story that brings home the worth of an individual's life. A despondent man wishes he had never been born, and a stranger grants him that wish. Then, when he sees the world as it would have been had he never been born, he realizes how precious and beautiful life is.

3. *The Secret Garden,* by Frances Hodgson Burnett (HarperTrophy, reprinted 1998): This is a tiny treasure of a book about how a garden can sweeten the sourest of natures. If you enjoyed this story as a kid, you'll cherish it as an adult; it is a gentle reminder to renew and refresh yourself.

4. *Illusions,* by Richard Bach. This book is about an aircraft, a writer, and a mechanic — but actually, it's about how to live and love. To me, it is literal proof of the adage "books give you wings." Read it when you're feeling low; your spirits will soar in no time. Long afterward, you'll still feel the echoes of Bach's life-enhancing messages.

• Breathe deeply. The simple act of drawing in a slow, relaxed breath is immensely calming. As you inhale, picture yourself imbibing joy. Expel the negativity and stress from within as you breathe out.

- Be aware of the present moment. The past is gone, and the future is a mystery. This moment is real. Enjoy it to the fullest.

- Meditation, the art of stillness, is a great source of healing for both mind and body. Choose a method that suits you, and set aside a few minutes a day to practice meditation, or *sadhana,* as Indian healers call it. To learn about Transcendental Meditation, a relaxation technique introduced by Maharishi Mahesh Yogi, visit www.tm.org. If you enjoy walking meditation, read the book *The Long Road Turns to Joy,* by Thich Nhat Hanh (Parallax Press, 1996). This Buddhist monk and teacher awakens you to walking, presenting it as a sublime joy and a mystical experience. Yes, it is written in childlike, simple prose, but in the space of a few pages, the book contains the essence of meditation. A must-read whether or not you're an avid walker.

Afterword

I wanted this book to be like a good friend who puts her arm around you, and says, "What do you need to feel your best? A cup of hot chocolate? A massage? A babysitter so you can take a nap?"

More than simply asking about your well-being, though, I wanted this book to offer you some irresistible ways to attract more calm, contentment, and cheerfulness into your life. I picked out the most pleasurable tips I could find and sprinkled them on these pages for you, like posies in a garden.

But don't think of these things as more items in your to-do list. In this garden of ideas, you are invited purely to be delighted! You don't have to stop and smell every flower, or adopt every suggestion you read here; if you feel inspired and excited when you read a certain tip I've given you, it's yours to enjoy. Just as a butterfly, charmed by a nectar-rich flower, stops awhile to sip; seek out the ideas that appeal to you, and allow yourself a moment of bliss, but don't be afraid to skip around.

Perhaps that is the most important message I can give you: Your bliss matters. As a woman, you're naturally inclined to and expected to take care of others first, but don't burn yourself out in the process. Realize, instead, that the more you look after yourself, the more meaningfully you'll be able to care about others. A refreshed and happy you will naturally be a nicer, more nurturing you. Better still, come home to a delightful truth: you deserve to feel good *just because it feels good.*

Once you believe that, the rest is easy. All you have to do is play with the suggestions in this book, try out one or a few at a time, make them your own, even share them with friends. Pretty soon you'll be creating new recipes for a delicious life.

You are the measure of this book's success. If, in the madness of modern life, I have cajoled you to linger awhile and sip some feel-good tea, or persuaded you to take a sunny view of life on a rainy day, then I have received my highest acclaim, my best review.

From the bottom of my heart, I wish you thousands of radiant, restful days to come.

Notes

Chapter 1
Joie de Vivre: How to Enjoy and Energize the Body You Inhabit

Epigraph: Norman O. Brown, *Love's Body* (New York: Vintage Books, 1967). American philosopher Norman O. Brown was born in 1913.

1. Howard Fast, "A Writer's Real Worth is Inside," in *Chicken Soup for the Writer's Soul: Stories to Open the Heart and Rekindle the Spirit of Writers,* edited by Jack Canfield (Deerfield Beach, Fla.: Health Communications, 1999).

Chapter 2
Nourishment: How to Savor the Bounteous Flavors of Health

Epigraph: Ralph Borsodi, *Flight from the City: An Experiment in Creative Living on the Land* (New York: Harper & Row Publishers, 1933). Robert Borsodi (1886–1977) was an author and philosopher.

1.   Donna Leahy, *Morning Glories: Recipes for Breakfast, Brunch, and Beyond from an American Country Inn* (New York: Rizzoli International Publications, Inc., 1996).

2.   Tom Colicchio, *Think Like a Chef* (New York: Clarkson Potter, 2000).

Chapter 3
Beauty: How to Be Lovelier — Inside and Out

Epigraph: Richard Brinsley Sheridan (1751–1816) was an Irish dramatist and politician.

1.   H. Jackson Brown, Jr., *Life's Little Instruction Book: 511 Suggestions, Observations, and Reminders on How to Live a Happy and Rewarding Life* (Nashville, Tenn.: Rutledge Hill Press, 1991).

2.   Sylvia Plath, *The Bell Jar* (London: Faber & Faber, 1963).

Chapter 4
Sanctuary: How to Make Your House a Home

Epigraph: Charles Dickens, *The Life and Adventures of Martin Chuzzlewit* (London: Chapman and Hall, 1844). Charles Dickens (1812–1870) was a British novelist and journalist.

1.   Cambridge Dictionaries (www.dictionary.cambridge.org).

Chapter 5
Love: How to Nurture Your Relationships

Epigraph: Leo Tolstoy, *War and Peace* (New York: Viking, 1982). Leo Tolstoy (1828–1910) was a Russian novelist.

1.   Richard Bach, *Illusions: The Adventures of a Reluctant Messiah* (New York: Dell Publishing, 1994).

2.   Sandy Sheehy, *Connecting: The Enduring Power of Female Friendships* (New York: William Morrow, 2000).

3. Bret Nicholaus and Paul Lowrie, *The Mom and Dad Conversation Piece* (New York: Ballantine Books, 1997).

4. Rabindranath Tagore, "The Judge," in *The Crescent Moon* (New York: The Macmillan Co., 1915).

5. Kahlil Gibran, *The Prophet* (New York: Alfred A. Knopf, 1923).

6. Ogden Nash, *Marriage Lines: Notes of a Student Husband* (Boston: Little, Brown, 1964).

Chapter 6
Repose: How to Relax and Revive Your Body and Mind

Epigraph: Indira Gandhi (1917–1984), quoted in *People,* June 30, 1975, was a politician and the prime minister of India.

1. Cambridge Advanced Learner's Dictionary, www.dictionary.cambridge.org.

2. Emily Dickinson, *The Complete Poems of Emily Dickinson* (Boston: Little, Brown, 1960), verse 254.

3. Lois Levy, *Undress Your Stress: 30 Curiously Fun Ways to Take Off Tension* (Naperville, Ill.: Sourcebooks, Inc., 1999).

Chapter 7
Bliss: How to Be Simply, Spiritually Happy

Epigraph: George Gissing (1857–1903) was a British novelist.

1. Louise Driscoll, "Hold Fast Your Dreams," in *Favorite Poems Old and New,* edited by Helen Ferris (New York: Doubleday & Company, 1957).

2. Allan Luks, *The Healing Power of Doing Good: The Health and Spiritual Benefits of Helping Others* (Lincoln, Neb.: Iuniverse.com books, 2001).

3. Jon Kabat-Zinn, *Wherever You Go, There You Are: Mindfulness Meditation in Everyday Life* (New York: Hyperion Books, 1995).

4. Rabindranath Tagore, *Rabindranath Tagore: An Anthology*, edited by Krishna Dutta and Andrew Robinson (New York: Griffin, 1999). Indian poet Rabindranath Tagore (1861–1941) received the Nobel Prize in literature in 1913.

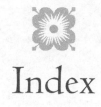

Index

About the Author

*L*ife, as Shubhra Krishan lives it, is one desperate deadline after another. She has reported for prime-time network news to an audience of 400 million viewers across India, and she's been an editor for *Cosmopolitan Magazine's* India edition. Currently, she works as Editorial Director for a Chicago-based company that produces films and television shows on health and entertainment. In short, she's the girl next door — who'd love to let her hair down and put her feet up more often.

In addition to writing about health and lifestyle topics for American magazines and Websites, Shubhra is now working on her first novel. She lives with her husband, Hemant, and son, Harshvardhan, in Colorado Springs.